MAGNET THERAPY

My 'Oscar' speech!

I need to thank several people, without whom
I would never have been able to write this book.

In the USA
To Lee Moore who first bullied me into placing a magnet on my body.
To Monica and Donna who taught me Magnet Therapy was not just
Mumbo Jumbo, and lastly but most of all to Jim Souder, whose
knowledge and devotion to Magnet Therapy convinced me this was a
truly remarkable and valuable new tool in healthcare.

In the UK
To my son Daniel and my Mother for just - being there.

Gloria Vergari MCMA

First Published in Great Britain in 2002 by
Norstar Biomagnetics International Limited,
Unit 4 Pipers Court, Berkshire Drive,
Pipers Way, Thatcham RG19 4ER

ISBN 0 9544262 0 7

Text ©2002 Gloria Vergari MCMA
Design and typesetting Milestone Strategic Design Ltd
Cover image Powerstock Ltd
Double Blind Studies provided by Coghill Research
Laboratories, Pontypool

Gloria Vergari is hereby identified as the author of this
work in accordance with Section 77 of the Copyright,
Design and Patents Act 1988

The contents of this book are for information only and are
intended to assist readers in identifying symptoms and
conditions they may be experiencing. The book is not
intended to be a substitute for taking proper medical
advice and should not be relied upon in this way. Always
consult a qualified doctor or health practitioner. The
author and publisher cannot accept responsibility for
illness arising out of the failure to seek medical advice
from a doctor.

WARNING: If you use pacemakers, defibrulators, insulin
pumps, or you are pregnant, DO NOT use magnetic therapy.

CONTENTS

PREFACE

Magnet Therapy by Gloria Vergari MCMA

Gloria Vergari is one of the first magnet therapists in England to be accredited by the Complementary Medical Association (CMA). Prior to that she studied magnet therapy under Jim Souder in America, one of the leaders in the technology of biomagnetic therapy in the USA.

She has devoted the last six years to pushing forward this new frontier in health care. In that period she has worked with over 4000 patients.

Magnet Therapy is not:
- A miracle or the answer to everything
- To be used without a diagnosis
  (an understanding of your condition).
- To be used by persons using a pacemaker, defibrillators, insulin pumps or other electro-insulin devices.
- To be used by pregnant women.

Magnet Therapy is:
- Doctor recommended
- Clinically tested
- Safe & effective
- Re-useable
- A non-invasive drug free therapy
- Affordable

According to Dr Ken Wianko, a top American physician:
"Magnets are not magic. Their function is very simple. Magnet therapy helps the body regain its self-healing balance naturally, because each organ and cell in the body is influenced by magnetic fields. Cell regulation, tissue function and life itself are controlled by electromagnetic currents."

"I honestly believe that simply wearing a modern magnet is one of the easiest ways we can enhance our well-being and combat the unusual, and in some cases unnatural, demands of the 21st Century."
Gloria Vergari

INTRODUCTION

This book is intended to be a simple guide to help in the understanding of how this new and important therapy works. Once you have grasped the basics, it is easy to understand how magnetic fields can aid the body and bring the results we see daily with our patients.

Over the last two years, Magnet Therapy has become a major talking point in the press and media and many of you are asking the following questions:

'Why have I only recently heard of it?'

Where did it come from?

Is it safe?

How should I use it?

In order to answer these questions I will take you on a fascinating journey that could change the way you approach healthcare.

In today's society the western world has come to believe, that most of us will live to our eighties or nineties. So when we, or our loved ones, don't achieve that ripe old age we almost feel slighted, as if we were cut short and cheated. Well 'good for us'. However, with this long lease on life comes the realisation that the NHS cannot and will not be there for every ache and pain – which means we will have to become familiar with ways of healing and maintaining our own bodies.

The general trend is to look for more natural ways of doing so. Over the last few years, the public both in the UK and throughout the world are opening up to complementary and alternative medicine, actively searching for non-intrusive, drug free and above all safe methods that are known to work. We are entering a new era in self-managed health care, and 'soft' medical alternatives are increasingly preferred over drugs and surgery whenever possible.

Magnet therapy is all of the above, and more. In this book we will attempt to explain how magnets effect changes in our health and well-being, and answer some of your questions, simply and frankly.

THE VALUE OF MAGNETIC FIELDS AND ENERGY

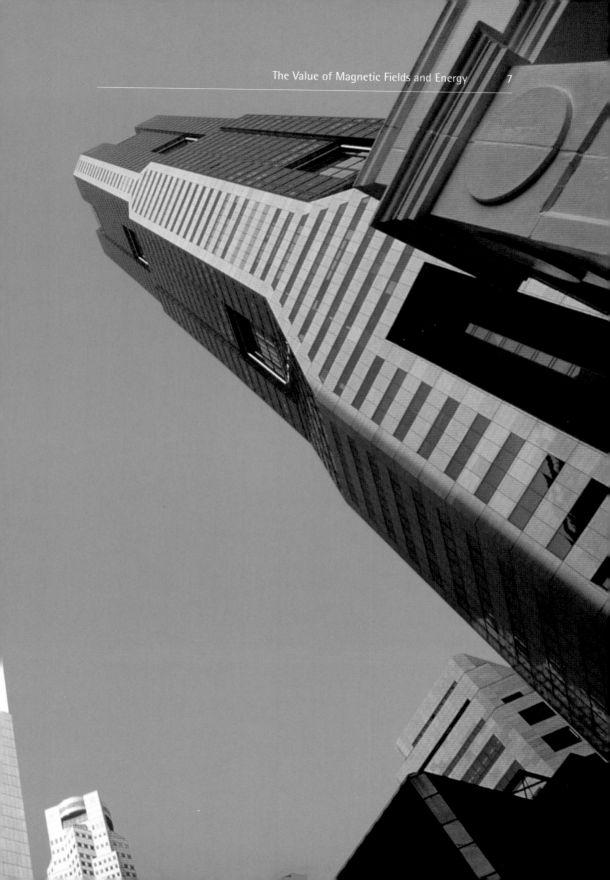

THE VALUE OF MAGNETIC FIELDS AND ENERGY

The universe, as Douglas Adams says in The Hitchhiker's Guide to The Galaxy, '...is big, it's very big'.

It is; think of all those planets, moons and stars out there, just hanging around in space. What is it that keeps them up in their own particular place and not crashing down into each other? It is gravity and magnetic fields continually pulling and opposing and holding the planets in their appointed place or orbits.

The Earth is in fact a giant magnet. Since the breakthrough theories of Einstein and other physicists we now have terms for the four forces which give and maintain order on our planet and in the universe: the weak nuclear force, the strong nuclear force, gravity, and the electromagnetic field.

The earth, mankind, animals, cells, atoms – life itself – are exposed to, and charged with, terrestrial magnetic fields. Every cell in our body has some energy or force flowing through it. To quote Shakespeare, not only are we "such stuff that dreams are made of" but we are also made up from the dust of ancient stars. Isn't that a lovely thought to hang onto as we are fighting the rush-hour crowds?

Attraction

When we are attracted to someone and say they have a magnetic personality or that there is some type of 'chemistry' happening, we are right – each of us gives off greater or lesser energies at slightly different strengths. A few of us with a naturally high output can become healers. The rest of us can now do the same to our bodies by utilising therapeutic magnets.

Remember the old cliché 'opposites attract'? The fact is that opposites are dynamic, creating change, pushing us ever forward. Positive and negative, yin and yang, hot and cold, dark and light, the moon, sun and earth are working towards our well-being. This wonderful energy field we were born into is crucial – indeed vital for our health.
Put simply, that means we are receiving less energy from the terrestrial magnetic fields that we readily obtained by living and working outside, in what was to us our natural environment. These changes are major; they have occurred in a relatively short space of time, not giving mankind enough time to evolve and adapt physiologically. Our buildings do insulate us from the health-giving elements we need. Consider the subtle changes that have occurred in a couple of generations: - we no longer walk barefoot on the earth, earn our living outside in the field or live in natural buildings made of wood and mud (all materials that contain and are conductive to magnetic fields, allowing them IN to our living environment). Isn't it true that most of us in the western world commute everywhere in metal capsules (cars, trains or plane). It is apparent to all of us, that the way we live has altered dramatically in the last century alone – chiefly with the advent of the industrial revolution and electricity in both our workplace and in our homes.

Modern pollution in terms of additives to our food and water supplies combined with the electrical waves we are surrounded by on a daily basis, bombard our bodies causing a new type of stress to our systems. Radio waves, microwaves, mobile phones, electric fields from overhead cables, and even our own home lighting and power for household appliances are present surrounding us.

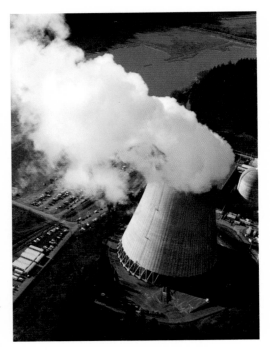

This cocktail of pollutants has depleted a significant amount of our own natural energy source. How much it has depleted our system is yet to be determined, but there is currently a lot of research going into the causes and triggers for such "modern" diseases as Magnetic Field Deficiency Syndrome (MFDS), Multiple Sclerosis (MS) and most notably ME. (Myalgic Enchephalomyelitis or Chronic Fatigue Syndrome).

Dr Nakagawa's recent research in Universities in Japan has helped to establish the concept of 'Magnetic Field Deficiency Syndrome'

He maintains that any changes in the Earth's magnetic field will negatively impact on the human body and function. Scientists know that the Earth is naturally loosing its magnetic field and this, combined with lifestyle changes, leads Nakagawa to maintain that this loss has resulted in a variety of disorders including neck and shoulder tension, headaches, lassitude, chest pains, lumbago, insomnia and constipation. Lethargy and constipation? Can magnets really help with that? "Right, sell me London Bridge whilst you're about it". I believe good quality Magnet Therapy can help to compensate us.

CASE STUDY

Roger Coghill

Roger Coghill, one of Britain's most noted researchers in the area of energy fields and medicine, tells us how metals react when placed in an electrical field.

He uses a particular case study to demonstrate:
He noted how a patient suffering from ME slept in a brass bed. At the back of this metal headboard was a double electric socket feeding two bedside lamps and a clock/radio, which were naturally kept switched on, merrily transmitting small amounts of electrical waves all through the night.

Roger immediately re-positioned her bed, removed the appliances, and told his patient to use a normal old-fashioned alarm clock and rely on her overhead lights. The patient quickly saw improvements in her health and strength.

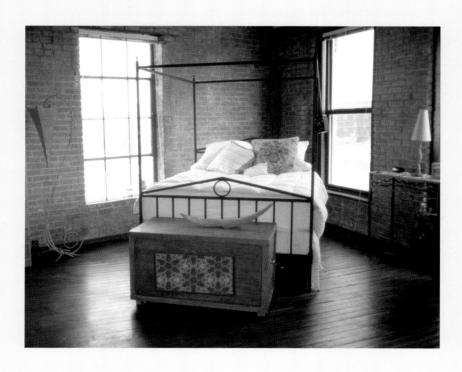

All of us have been brought up taking the benefits of electricity for granted. None of us would dream of turning back the clock and living without electric power, but it may have taken a toll on our system, and we may have to become somewhat clearer and more discerning in how we use it if we want to improve and maintain good health. For instance, I have now made simple changes in my household, small things, such as putting my dishwasher and washing machine on - when I leave the kitchen area or at bedtime. Why? Because I do not want their particular energy output to interfere with and deplete mine.

I have also taken my bedside lamps away and rely on normal overhead lighting. After all I did not grow up with bedside lamps and how much effort it is really to go over to the wall and switch the lights off? As I said, small changes, but why not try and see how your body can recover over a period.

My concern for our children

If we look at youngsters' rooms, it is quite disturbing to see the amounts of sockets, cables and screens that surround them when they sleep, and usually in reasonably confined spaces. Should we take a look at those consequences on their future health? I believe we should. It really does concern me that during these vital growing years we are allowing so much electrical pollution to impact on their maturing systems.

Again, Roger Coghill's recent research in the UK, which studies the effects of EMF's and RF/MW (radio waves/micro waves) radiation is finally drawing the attention of relevant bodies who may at some point advise us on the simple precautions we can now take when raising young children. Hopefully educating us in ways to reduce some of the triggers, which may add to the increase in cases of sudden infant death syndrome (SIDS).

What would I do if I were starting a family today?

I would observe some simple precautions in decorating my infant's room, making it as free from electrical stimuli as I could possibly make it. According to Roger – all humans are born premature – In as much as our brains are not fully myelinated at birth. This means that, for the first year of our life our brains do not have the fatty insulating covering that myelination later provides. The young infant at this stage is more susceptible to RF/MW frequencies. So try to keep them at bay. Use overhead lights – not bedside ones. No power points by their cribs, and one last thing, if you have to use a baby sound monitor – Do NOT place it by baby's head. If you need to use one, place it by the feet or thereabouts.

You see, once we begin to see ourselves as an energy source, we want to encourage our normal frequency to have full range and not be interrupted by other frequencies that are at slight variants with our own. If something is picking up and transmitting sound – there are RW/MW's around. I have been told that you have to have a license in Germany to own a microwave. Enough said!

None of this is aimed at scare tactics or dreaded warnings of doom, on the contrary, I love this modern world and most of what is has to offer, let's use it. But use it wisely. And MOST of all – let's protect and ensure the most incredible machine we walk around in for our time on Earth – is nurtured!

According to NASA the earth has lost over 14% of it's magnetic field in the last 200 years alone, and adding the two things together you can see that we may be functioning slightly under par - our "batteries" may have had the edge taken off them.

Strangely enough two places on Earth are said to have a higher magnetic reading than others, one is Sedona in the USA, the other is Lourdes in France, both famous centres of healing.

THE HISTORY OF MAGNETIC THERAPY

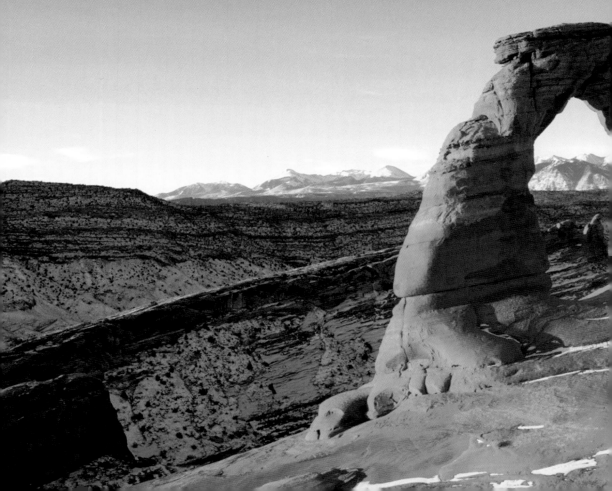

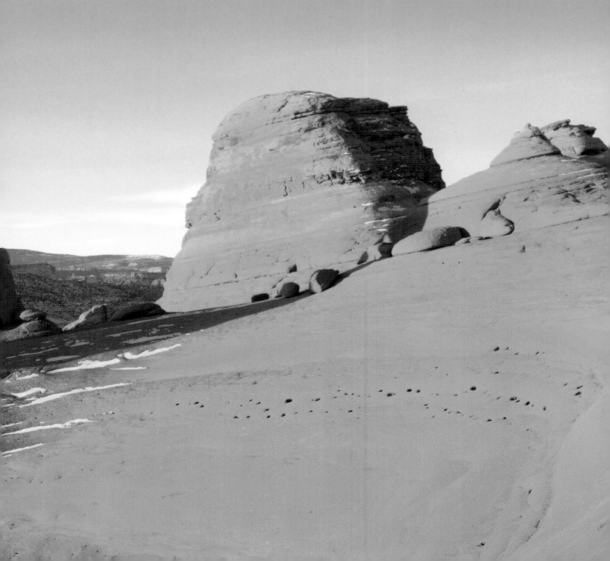

THE HISTORY OF MAGNETIC THERAPY

Magnetic Fields and their effects on life on earth has been recognised by scientists for a thousand years. Now doctors are coming to realise its vital necessity in maintaining our health.

A Short History of Medicine

2000 B.C. Here, eat this root.

A.D.1000 That root is heathen. Here, say this prayer.

A.D.1850 That prayer is superstition. Here, drink this potion.

A.D.1940 That potion is snake oil. Here, swallow this pill.

A.D.1985 That pill is ineffective. Here, take this antibiotic.

A.D.2000 That antibiotic is artificial. Here, eat this root.

In other words, whenever possible or practical, we are turning back to remedies found in nature.

In China

4000 years ago, there were no known writings relating to medicine or health care. However, in China there was a well-developed system in place. It was based on the understanding that good health depended on the circulation of vital energies. These energies would follow prescribed pathways through the body.

This internal strength or energy was called Qi (chi).
Most of us have heard of yin and yang, this is the understanding derived from two opposing influences that balance each other out (remember positive and negative). The Chinese healers presumed that when the influences of yin and yang were out of harmony

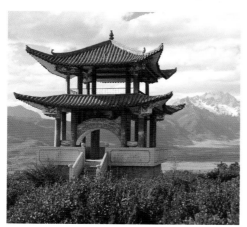

the natural flow of Qi was blocked, causing an un-natural balance in the body resulting in illness.

The Chinese placed a great deal of emphasis on the importance of the Qi (energy) flowing unimpaired through the body.

The first major work on healing was called The Emperor's Book of Internal Medicine. This book recorded and described how imbalances could be corrected by the use of what we now know to be acupuncture and the use of magnetic stones. The Chinese went on to explain how key points in the body related to different organs and energy lines.

In Egypt

Egyptian physicians were using lodestones (magnets) for a variety of conditions. Queen Cleopatra herself wore a small magnet in an amulet on her forehead to preserve her youth.

We know today how right she was, but how did she know this?

At the back of the forehead lies the pineal gland; this is quite small (about the size if a pine nut). The pineal is home to melatonin, which is secreted by the gland at night. Melatonin is also a powerful antioxidant and is now being hailed as the 'youth hormone' due to it's potential for cell repair and anti-aging. Did Cleopatra know something that we are now re-discovering? Probably! Today, instead of hanging an amulet on our forehead, we can simply sleep on a magnetic pillow pad to achieve the same result. It is like having an eight-hour, oxygen-rich beauty treatment while we sleep.

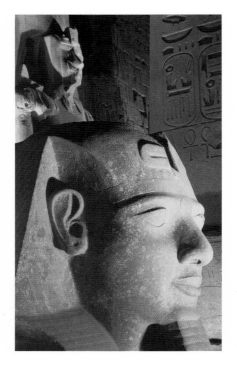

Melatonin in pill form has also become very popular as a sleep aid and is used widely for jetlag and regulating sleep patterns.

Again, sleeping on a magnetic pad will encourage the pineal gland to naturally secrete melatonin and thus secure the same result as the pill.

In Greece

Thales, a Greek philosopher who lived in the 7th century, said, 'All things are full of Gods'. He made this remark when noting that if amber, (a fossilised tree resin), was rubbed with wool it would pick up light objects such as straw or feathers. Somehow it 'attracted' them.

The Greeks were also the first people to understand the properties of magnetite (lodestone) and how these grey stones could attract nails and other items made of iron. Thales thought that magnetite 'has soul because it attracts iron'. They saw these things as magic from the gods. Our ancestors simply observed the effects these special stones could have in healing and worked with them believing the gods used them to intervene and help mankind. They watched and observed through the centuries, noting many useful ways of healing with plants and stones that nature had given us. Sadly, many of these findings have been lost to us for centuries and some perhaps forever.

In Europe

We can then skip through the Dark Ages, but in passing we have to acknowledge the part played by Paracelcus (1493-1541) in furthering our understanding of magnets and note the part he foresaw them playing in healing both in humans and animals. Later, during the glorious reign of Elizabeth I, where it was widely reported that her personal physician Dr William Gilbert (1540-1600) would treat strangulated hernia (twisted hernia) by using iron fillings. Dr Gilbert would have the filings baked into a cake. Legend says he then fed the cakes to his patient, and waited for them to be partially digested. By placing a lodestone (magnet) over the lower stomach area he would untwist the hernia.
How about that for non-invasive surgery! Dr Gilbert also believed that whatever strange force existed in magnets, it was the key to life.

Just look at Michelangelo's breathtaking painting on the ceiling of the Sistine Chapel. It shows Adam being animated by God with what appears to be the "spark of life." It is certain - that energy medicine will lead us to the next generation of healing?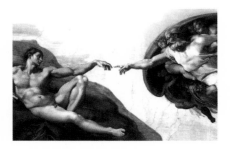

In the 18th & 19th centuries many noted scientists and physicians experimented with magnetic fields and electricity. The knowledge and the materials they had were pretty crude, but they had valiant stabs at understanding things we are becoming more and more aware of.

One of these young academic doctors was an Austrian, called Franz Mesmer. Today he is somewhat ridiculed as the 'quack' who used to hypnotise his patients. Hence, the word 'mesmerise'. Mesmer was in fact a brilliant young man who studied mathematics, the law and medicine. His doctoral thesis dealt with the effects of gravitational fields and cycles on human health. He was ridiculed and derided by the medical establishment in Vienna, and hounded out of the city. Over the years he practiced medicine, using his knowledge of magnetic fields, and patients from all over Europe soon flocked to him for treatment. His popularity grew by word of mouth and he became one of the most successful and controversial men in Paris. The medical community was, as always conservative; they thought him a hoax and all the cures he achieved to be due to his power of suggestion. In other words he 'mesmerised' them.

If only Mesmer were alive today to see the modern magnets, their strengths and flexibility, he would be completely vindicated and respected for the visionary and scientist he was.

Today Tibetan monks still use large lodestones around the head for clarity of thought, and to improve the concentration and learning capacity of their young monks during training.

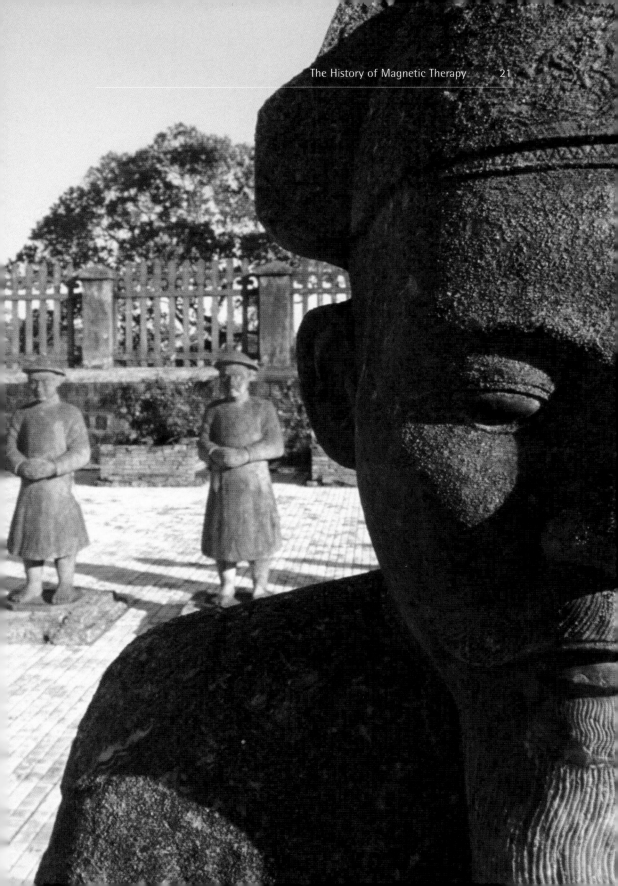

MODERN OR THERAPEUTIC MAGNETS

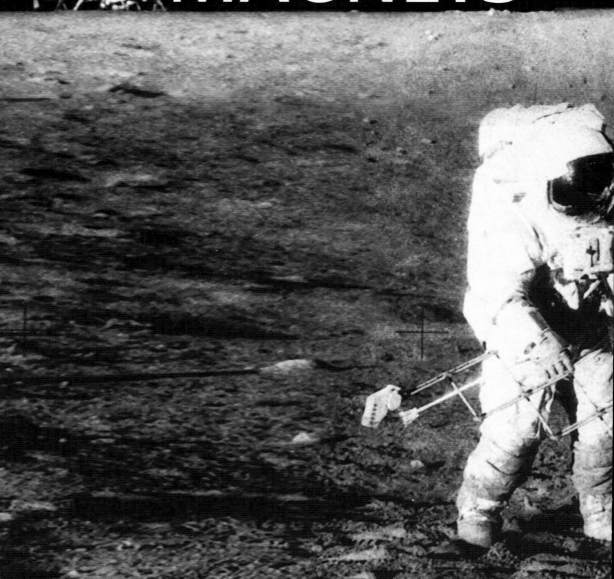

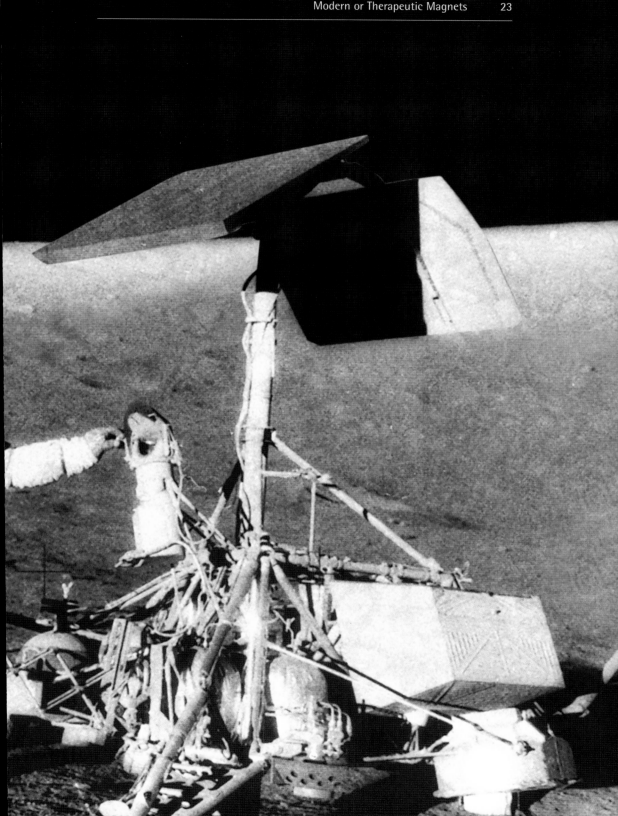

MODERN OR THERAPEUTIC MAGNETS

It is said that we owe modern 'medical' magnets to the space industry. Certainly they played a major part in developing the materials we now use in magnet and biomagnetic therapies. It was also responsible for introducing to a wider audience the vital role the earth's magnetic field has on the human body, and in maintaining its full potential.

When man first ventured into space in the 1960s, we understood the need to provide him with a safe, reliable spacecraft. The astronaut was given a life-supporting suit and went through a thorough training programme to withstand the mental and physical challenges we understood he would encounter. He was then sent off into the great unknown, and the space agencies made sure the back up on earth was of the highest calibre.

We know just how successful, both the Americans and Russians were in this enterprise. We were amazed and delighted to see the astronauts return from their pioneering endeavours, tired but safe. However, it was determined by constant monitoring from earth during their relatively short time in space that the men were losing bone density; their immune systems were being affected and they were experiencing calcium deficiency. After the initial space flights it was necessary for the astronauts to be placed into isolation for several weeks upon their return. During this quarantine period following a flight, it became clear that the physiological changes that occurred were partly a result of man leaving the Earth's magnetic field. Their systems were under stress and not able to function properly. As I mentioned before - this magnetic energy field is something we were born into, as a species we evolved in it.

Modern medicine now understands how essential this natural energy source is to life. Without it our bodies suffer. We lose the energy (Qi) to produce the normal level of bodily activity, and most importantly our ability to repair ourselves.

What to do?
Whether it was the Russian or American space programme that first came to understand the nature of the problem is not quite certain, but it was decided to place large magnetic blocks inside each spacecraft. This did begin to alleviate the medical problems faced by the astronauts, but the increased load affected the fuel efficiency of the crafts on take-off. Therefore another solution had to be found.

At this point we are told the space agencies approached outside businesses and asked them to develop extremely high-powered magnets that were lightweight. This they did, very successfully, and they came up with several of the materials that are now widely used in modern magnet-therapy.

To explain the breakthrough that was made in the technology I will use an example you can readily understand:
an industrial magnet that may hold a note on your refrigerator door is about -100 gauss (term used in calculating the strength of a magnet) – whilst a magnet we now use in health care, can be the same size and weight as that fridge magnet, and yet hold a magnetic strength of – 12,300 gauss.

What does this mean to us?
It means, lightweight, portable magnets that are strong enough to stimulate changes in the way our cells behave and react.

NOTE:
Today, when astronauts go into space they wear suits lined with flexible magnetic materials, and the spacecraft has a magnetic lining. Now, when they return from a flight, whether it is two days or two months they go straight from the craft and into a press conference. This is a good example of how important maintaining our magnetic balance can be in the way we function.

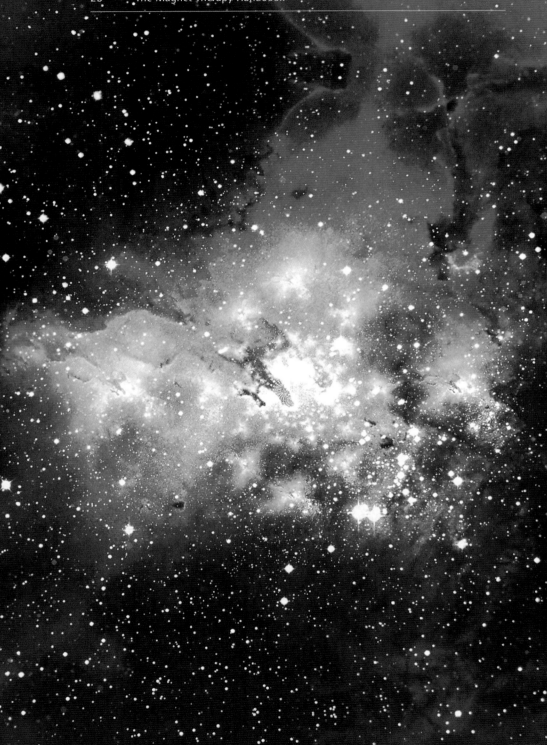

The Worldwide use of Magnets

Western countries tend to be dominated by a belief in pharmaceutical drugs. However, in countries where this is not the case and drugs are not automatically turned to, magnetic therapy is often the first line of approaching soft tissue damage. Countries such as Japan, Russia and China use them continually.

As we mentioned earlier, China has done so for the last 4000 years, but with today's materials and technology, we do not have to haul around a massive lodestone.

Over the last few years, countries such as Germany, and most recently the USA, are fast catching on to the benefits of this exceptional new modality. The USA in particular is now actively involved in research programmes to determine the most effective ways to use therapeutic magnets, driven largely by the American public's curiosity, as they have experienced the benefits and results. Hopefully, we will all gain a deeper insight into magnet therapy and other emerging forms of energy medicine.

It is a truly remarkable threshold we are on.

> We are changing the way we see ourselves, from simply 'organic man' – to a 'charged organic man' with our own amazing - energy pack. In fact we come with "Batteries included!"

HOW A SCEPTIC BECAME A BELIEVER

WEST SIDE STORY

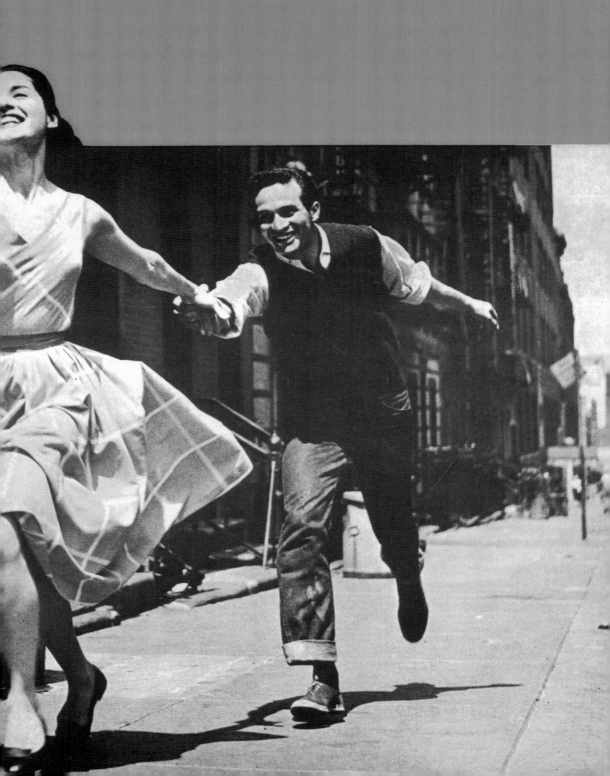

HOW
A SCEPTIC
BECAME A
BELIEVER

Thirty years ago I had a serious knee accident, when as a professional dancer in London I fell during one of the more active scenes in West Side Story. I was in a rehearsal class, and being a 'cocky soul', I decided to try the boy's dance, as the men's work was stronger, harder and far more challenging. It was during the 'COOL' routine that it happened, I was having a terrific time, spinning and leaping and really pushing myself – then I jumped, missed the landing – and FELL. I fell, and heard several bones crack, so did the guys around me! Yet, being the true trooper that I was, I managed to hobble off stage and get myself down to Charring Cross Hospital.

Over the next nine months I was cut, stitched screwed and finally plastered back together. The bones finally mended, and I did go back to dancing. I even managed to work at the Moulin Rouge in Paris for a season; doing their world famous Can-Can. But the ligaments in my damaged knee let me know they weren't happy. Tearing the same knee in a skiing accident a few years later, did not do much to help the situation, but given a sporting chance, the human body does like to repair itself, whenever possible, and my knee did, at least partially.

Whilst not too bad for most activities and sports, my knee does not like concrete, and whilst jogging one evening in 1997 with friends in North Carolina, it gave out on me. I was suddenly in severe pain and could not walk on it. I asked my friends to book an appointment the following day with a local physiotherapist. This injury was an old pal – it had reared its head periodically and I knew I needed a few sessions of ultra-sound and some anti-inflammatory pills for a couple of weeks.

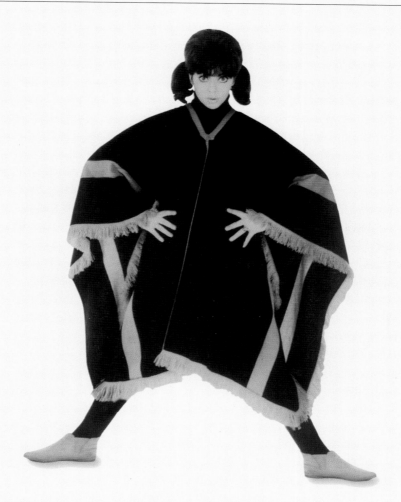

One of my friends handed me a knee wrap and said, "here try this until morning". I asked what it was and when he told me it had magnets in it, I politely told him to get lost. Some new gimmick from America, I thought! He insisted I try it. I refused and so on until he wore me down and I agreed to keep it on until I saw the physio in the morning. The following morning I got up, took the wrap off to shower, and low and behold there was not a trace of inflammation in my leg. I gingerly handed it back to Lee and said, "Thanks." I thought it was interesting, but would not believe the wrap had anything to do with it – I wanted to believe my knee had just spontaneously healed. In thirty years it had never done so before, but a magnet? Well really! I dismissed the idea.

Two weeks later, whilst moving a table in their house I tore a muscle in my shoulder. Obviously somewhere in my deep unconscious I had remembered the magnets, because I asked them if I could stick the knee wrap over my shoulder. They laughed, said I would look like The Hunchback of Notre Dame, and Lee promptly took me to meet Donna, the magnet therapist they had bought their knee wrap from. After a brief consultation, I was told that all I needed for my torn muscle was a powerful neodymium magnet. It was the size and weight of a 2p coin, but had the horsepower of a tank. Donna simply attached it to my deepest point of pain using a medical tape. Within 24 hours the pain was gone and I had full mobility in arm and shoulder. As you can imagine, this now had my full attention. Over the years I had suffered enough injuries dancing, teaching aerobics and skiing to know something was happening inside my body; tissue did not usually respond like this. I went back to the therapist and she spent time with me, explaining the basics of what happened when a magnetic field is applied to the body, and how this new method of healing was sweeping the USA. In - spite of drug companies trying to discredit it, the public knew it worked and millions of Americans were now successfully using magnets.

By this time I was becoming extremely interested in the science behind Magnetic Field Therapy and Donna advised me to go down to Raleigh, North Carolina, and talk to one of the leaders in the research and development of biomagnetics, Jim Souder. Jim is respected throughout the community as a man of great integrity and a true innovator in the field. I went to Jim's clinic and stayed in his house and studied with him and his wife Judi for several months. They opened up a new world to me, and on my return to England I decided to spend time testing magnets. I did so; on friends, family, neighbours – and their animals. No one was safe around me, I stuck magnets here, I placed them there! For six months I cautiously (and sceptically) watched and monitored my friends, and slowly I came to understand how truly amazing were the results I was witnessing. I took a deep breath and decided to throw caution and money to the wind. This meant giving up a career that had been very lucrative for 17 years in order to pursue this subject.

Background

Following the death of my husband in England in 1981, I stuck my long-suffering 10 year old son, Daniel under my arm and headed for the USA to start a new life. Shortly after I arrived in America, I set up a consulting business in Los Angeles working and advising leading US furniture manufacturers on how to use the best of Italian design and modify it for the American market. I sourced product from all over Italy and the Far East. I was my own boss, I travelled the world and it was extremely rewarding, as only the USA can be. The industry had fed, nourished and indulged Daniel and me for 17 good years, and I had a very good reputation in the trade. Then I strapped a knee wrap on my knee.

Suddenly, I was now about to give this all up to bring 'Magnet Therapy' to England. Daniel thought me mad!

Not to be distracted I decided to liquidate an entire warehouse full of furniture just to focus on my new evangelical quest. How could I not - I began to study everything I came across concerning the therapeutic use of magnets, and was continually amazed by what I read and saw. Six years on, and some 4000 patients later, I still find it hard to believe something this small and simple can actually be so effective and can deal with such a wide variety of conditions that I see every week. Usually these are the types of conditions that doctors have said, 'well there is nothing more I can do for you, keep on with the painkillers'. Later in this book you will read about some case studies, and see the letters our patients and customers send us. The overwhelming encouragement I received from the public was enough to keep me going during the cold, harsh initial years in the UK.

In England, there appeared to be no standards in place for magnet therapists, and by pure chance, I met Valerie Dargonne, a young woman who had been independently studying this field of energy medicine for years. We both had similar intentions and aims for the future of magnets in the UK. Both of us wanted to get this therapy taken seriously by medical and professional health care practitioners. Valerie and I wanted to establish some sort of intelligent guideline, and with this in mind we created a comprehensive training programme. Over several months Valerie developed our course and to date we have trained and accredited over 50 therapists, six doctors, and three dentists with more coming on board daily. We are the only school of magnet therapy to be accredited in the UK by The Complementary Medical Association.

I hope I can now share with you this simple therapy.

HOW DO MAGNETS WORK?

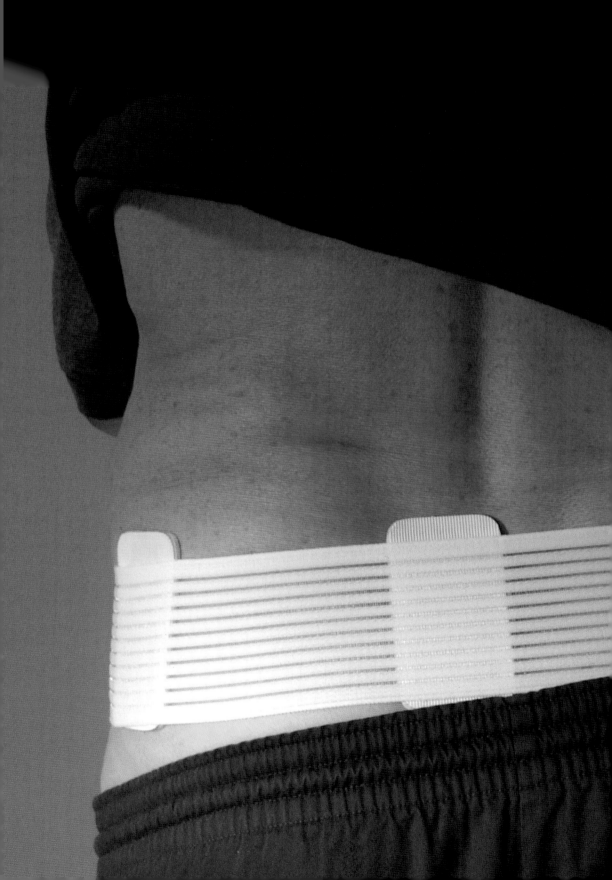

HOW DO MAGNETS WORK?

There is still much research and debate about how magnets work. Different theories have been claimed by manufacturers of magnetic products. I will point out the largely accepted views held by doctors and researchers.

EXTRACT FROM A DOUBLE BLIND STUDY
by St Pauls College of Vetinary Medicine USA 1995

> 'When a magnet is applied to the body muscles and soft tissue lengthen and relax, waves pass through the tissue and secondary currents are induced. When those currents clash with magnetic waves they produce impacting heat on electrons in the body cells. These impacting heats are very effective in the reduction of muscle swelling and pain. Movement of haemoglobin in the blood vessels is accelerated, this has been observed in both thermographic and nuclear medicine studies, while calcium, cholesterol and lactic acid deposits in the blood are decreased. The fatigued blood is cleansed and circulation is increased.
>
> There is also significant evidence of a pain blocking mechanism in nerve fibres themselves when subjected to magnetic fields. Researchers have been able to shift the resting potential (thereby raising the required stimulus to pain) of nerve cells in the laboratory by 25% using the Norso Dynamag technology (Jim Souder's company). 'High strength magnets can cause anaesthesia, in the tissue, through a principal in physics called the Hall effect. A thermal impact that occurs within the cell, which can affect nerve signals'.

What does this all mean in lay terms?

Two vital things occur when a magnet is placed on the skin:

- First, the soft tissue will lengthen and help to relax down a muscle or ligament that is damaged or traumatised. It will work in an area and depth directly proportional to the type and strength of magnet used (forget the fridge one). Presuming you have one of the better magnets – I will give you the guide lines in the following chapter – you should be able to effect a change to a radius of between 3 – 5 inches around any one magnet and to a similar depth.

- Secondly, the tissue relaxes, oxygen and blood flow that has so far had restricted access to the damaged site is allowed in and is increased. We can see this by thermal imaging.

Normally an injured site, whether from arthritis, torn muscles or any other condition, will be surrounded by inflammation. This can comprise of lactic acids, calcium and other deposits. Basically the site is 'hot' with acidity. The increase in oxygen and blood flow brings with it increased alkaline. Acidity hates to be in an alkaline environment and this is where the body starts to generate its own healing abilities. Magnets merely encourage this in a truly dramatic way.

So, here we are - we have relaxed the tissue and, with increased blood flow, we have started to detoxify the area. Next, the thermal impact mentioned in the study above occurs inside the cell.

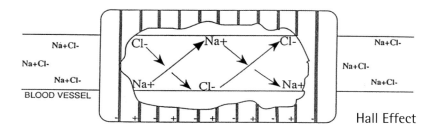

Hall Effect

CASE STUDY

Industrial Injury – Partially Severed Hand
Andy Burgess, Axbridge

My name is Andy Burgess; I'm 39 and a general builder. On the 7th April 1998 I was involved in an industrial accident, which resulted in my wrist being severely cut, and the doctors advised me I might lose my hand. All my tendons were severed, as were my arteries and veins. After many operations and over 250 internal stitches they managed to save my hand. Many months later I had 65% mobility but a great deal of pain. Every morning I woke with a 'clawed hand' and it took 20 minutes of exercise to release it.

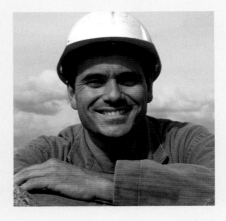

Some numbness still remained, and the hand was weak (I could not lift a kettle).

After using your magnetic link bracelet the 'clawing' stopped within days and I can honestly say that since I have been wearing it my wrist and fingers are now nearly normal. I can work again and lift anything up to 60lbs with it.

I would recommend these products to anyone without hesitation, and do, as I am living proof that these things work.

Keep up the good work.
A.S. Burgess,
Somerset March 2001

Andy has been back working regularly in the building trade ever since.

As the blood in our body continuously circulates it periodically comes close to the magnet placed on the skin above. The ions in the blood become agitated and are attracted to the magnet, atomic particles begin to spin inside the cell – they go into the Hall effect – and in doing so get 'switched on'.

By 'switching on' the body kicks in its own beta-endorphin (pain relieving) system.

So to recap, we expect magnet therapy to activate the following responses in the body:

1. Lengthen and relax tissue.

2. Begin the process of flushing out debris and inflammation from the site.

3. Kick in the body's own pain relieving system.

These are the key points you must understand about magnetic products if you wish to successfully treat yourself and your family. If you understand that the product works where it is placed you will not fall into the trap of buying a wristband to help with pain in your knee.
If a magnet is going to work for you, it can happen within hours when quality magnets are placed over the damaged area. Normally we expect to see improvements within 1 – 7 days, when you are directly treating the site of pain.

A wristband or sufficiently strong bracelet is fine if you have hand or wrist pain, or if you want to maximize your general health and encourage your body to detoxify. You will keep the bracelet in place for long periods, as it is easy to wear. But there is little point in relaxing and promoting blood flow to your wrist if your problem is your lower back!

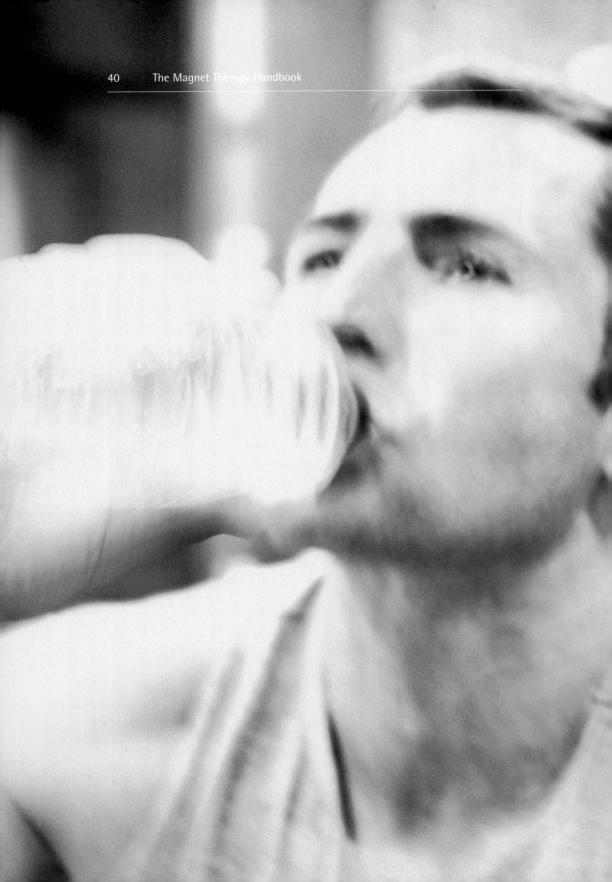

Wearing a magnet anywhere on the body will still have the same detoxifying effect on the blood, after a period of time. As I mentioned before – the agitation within the cells releases the debris that naturally clings to the walls.

One thing you must remember when you use magnet therapy and that is to drink at least 3 - 4 glasses of water a day. You need to flush out of your system the toxins that magnets are releasing from the cells. Coffee, tea (whether herbal or not), fruit juice are just not the same as water. The body treats them differently.

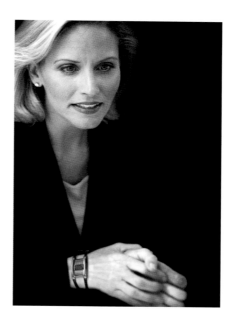

We are 75% water and we need to replenish the cells. Use, spring, mineral or tap, anything whatever you prefer – just WATER.

If your general health is good, and you have no immediate areas to be healed, then by all means wear a magnetic bracelet. It is the simplest most effective way to compensate for the man-made EMF pollutants that deplete our systems. A good magnetic bracelet will help to boost and support the body's own bio-energy system. Choose a 'North Pole' bracelet and make sure it is sufficiently strong to effect changes. My therapists and I all use bracelets. However, drinking water still applies!

Flush out the toxins that magnets release with water!

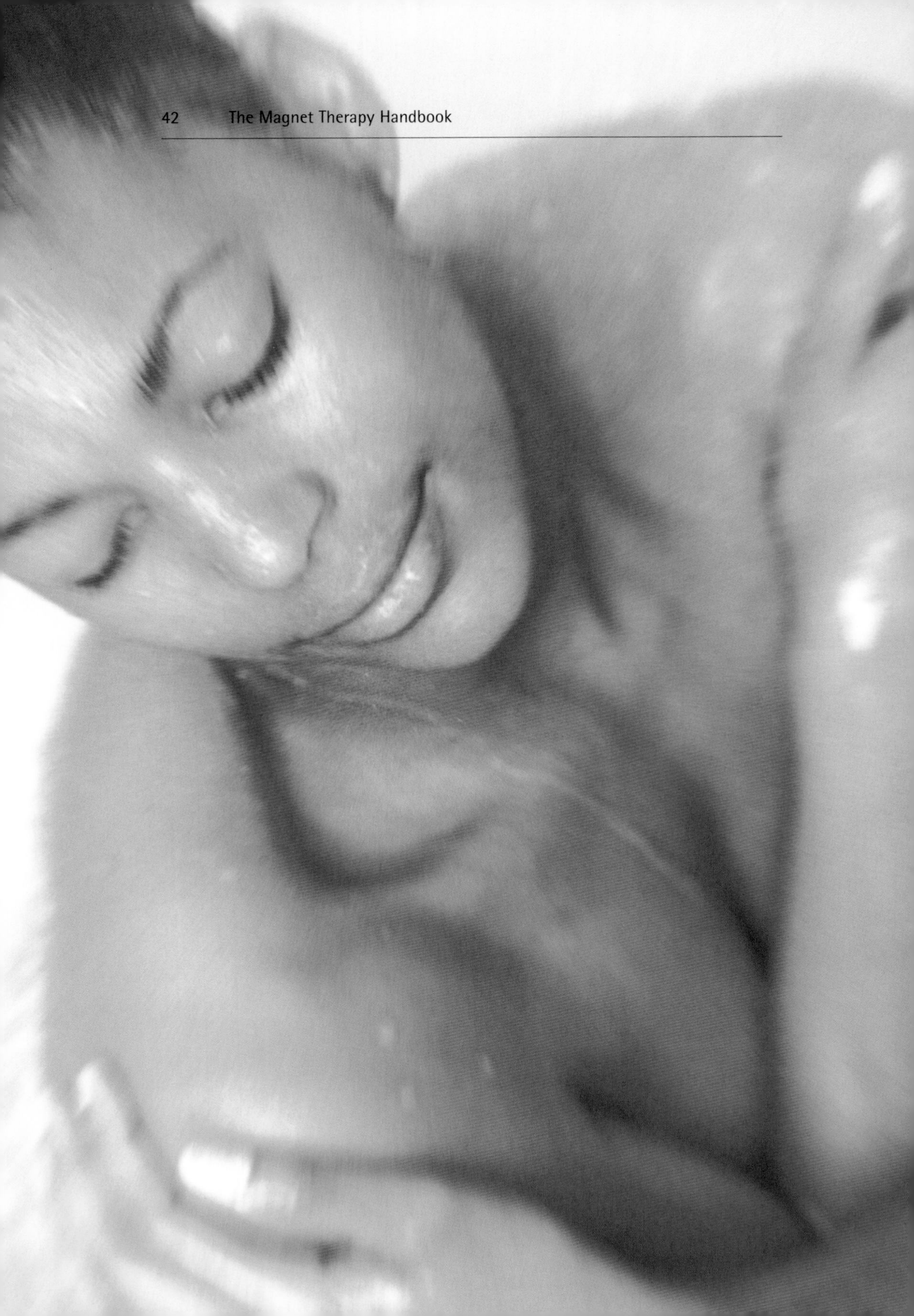

THE MAIN AREAS OF BENEFIT SEEN IN MAGNET THERAPY

- Helps alleviate pain and improves mobility of arthritic joints

- Eases stress, depression, promotes sound sleep

- Aids recovery of nerve sensation

- Aids recovery of torn ligaments, muscles and tendons

- Reduces bruising and swelling

- Speeds recovery in sports injuries

- Increases resistance to infection

- Improves circulation / body and extremity warming

- Helps removal of waste products from the blood i.e. lactic acids, calcium, cholesterol and fat deposits

- Increases energy and strength

- Speeds healing i.e. bone fractures

- Helps recovery or can prevent onset of R.S.I / Carpal Tunnel Syndrome

- Alleviates migraine and headaches

- Improves overall health

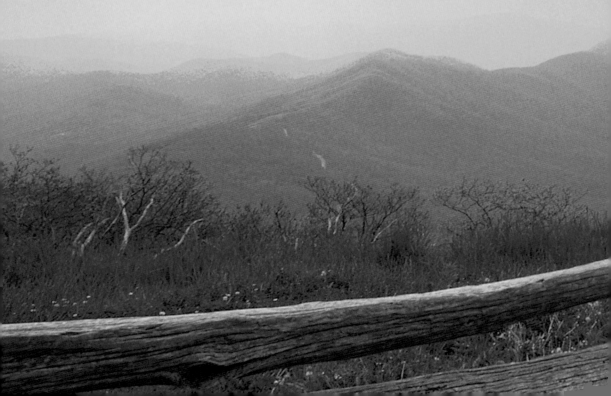

HEALING
WITH
MAGNETS

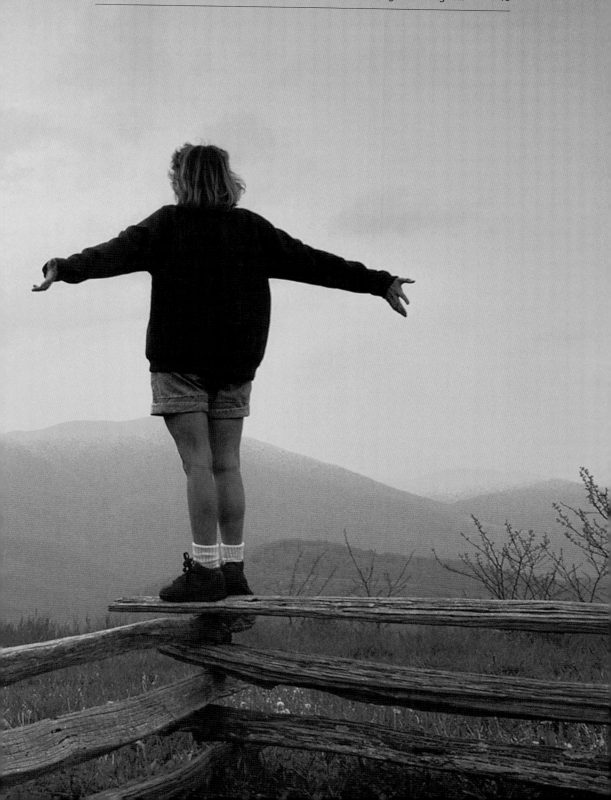

HEALING
WITH
MAGNETS

**Some interesting facts according to Dr Mark Atkinson MBBS
Author of WHOLE BODY HEALING.**

Although medical doctors and researchers remain sceptical as to the effectiveness of magnet therapy, recent research studies from major universities and medical colleges have shown the benefits of static magnet fields in relieving pain.

The Office of Alternative Medicine of the Institute of Health, Washington, D.C. awarded a million dollar grant in 1997 for the study of what has been, until now, largely an Eastern and European phenomenon. Medical use of magnets is reimbursable by private health care in 50 countries worldwide.

Baylor College of Medicine, USA. Dr Carlos Valbona in 1997 published a double blind study of 50 patients who suffered from muscular or arthritic pain. 76% of patients treated with static magnets reported significant improvement.

New York Medical College, N.Y. Dr Michael Weintraub, a clinical professor of neurology released a study in 1999 that showed he had significantly reduced foot pain in diabetics, by the use of magnetic innersoles in 9 out of 10 patients.

Vanderbilt University Medical Center, found that between 80%-90% of patients with pain related to sports injuries and accidents found relief after magnet treatment.

The Kouseikai Suzuki Hospital, Dr Shimoda in Japan, in double blind clinical studies showed that 83% of their patients with sleep related disorders benefited from the use of magnetic mattress pads.

One in three households in Japan sleeps on a magnetic mattress pad.

BUYER BEWARE

Before you buy your magnets – know how to select the one that is right for you.

Many people use magnets that are ineffective because they are simply not powerful enough. This can give magnet therapy a bad name.

MAGNETS DO WORK!

In the USA alone, the public are now spending over $500 million a year on magnet therapy, with a large portion of that money going on mattress pads. Worldwide the figure is growing at such a rate it is difficult to put a realistic figure on the sales. The rapidly growing markets are currently Israel, Germany and the UK.

Magnets can significantly help your body to help itself, but they must be the best quality and configuration of magnetic fields you can find.
My mantra: 'Not all magnets are created equal'

You just have to buy the best, and the best may not be the most expensive ones. Certainly I have seen some magnets that are on sale that are twice the price and half as strong as other reliable brands. As you will be largely self treating yourself and your family you must learn one or two key things in about determining the right product to buy.

Buy a magnet designed for your requirements. For example wrist magnet for wrist/hand conditions, a mattress pad for sleep disorders.

The next thing I want you to remember, is the term 'GAUSS RATING'. The gauss of a magnet determines it strength. There is a gauss rating at the centre (core) of the magnet and one at its surface.

NEODYMIUM – THE 'KING' OF MAGNETS

Neodymium magnets are made up of three metals: boron, ferrite and neodymium. Neodymium is a rare earth metal and it is expensive. The quantity of neodymium in the magnet directly affects the power of that magnet.

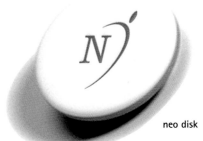

neo disk

Top quality neodymium's can have a CORE rating of 12,300 and a SURFACE gauss of 1,200. This magnet will have an impact of 3 – 6 inches on the skin both in radius and in depth of penetration.

The surface area of the magnet will also determine the penetration (i.e. 1/2" neodymium will have less penetration than a 1" neo although the strength is the same). A reliable supplier will know how to build an appropriate wrap for the area in question.

We call neodymiums 'permanent' magnets and they will hold their fields for up to 15 years.

These magnets should be used for most soft tissue damage as they are the ones likely to get the best results for places such as backs, knees hips, shoulders etc.

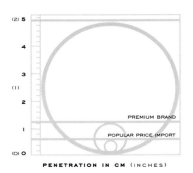

penetration comparison chart

I have seen some magnets with a core gauss of 400. The surface rating is barely anything and it would be lucky to penetrate 1/8". Some of these are 'exhausted' after a few days and the manufacturer suggests you throw them away.

Choosing a magnet is like buying a car. Go to a therapist or look for packaging you can trust. Make sure you understand what you are getting. Do NOT go for attractive packaging or advertisements. Read the information, ask the therapist or call the help line. If the packaging does not tell you the strength (GAUSS, surface and core) DO NOT BUY. Your results depend on it. The search for a good product does really pay off in the end.

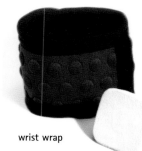

wrist wrap

It was neodymium magnets that enabled Silence of the Lambs star, Anthony Hopkins to finish a film on schedule. He had been in agony suffering from a frozen shoulder. To quote Mr Hopkins, "Magnets are the answer to my prayers. I suffered from terrible shoulder pain for years, so when I heard about magnet therapy, I jumped at the chance to try it. I just applied magnetic patches to my shoulder for a week or two, and I got so much relief from them I did not need them again for months. Magnets are truly wonderful."

FLEXIBLE MAGNETS

A less expensive magnet is a FLEXIBLE one. A flexible magnet is approximately 2,750 gauss at its core. This will have an impact on tissue of between 1" – 2". Flexible magnets are used for fingers, thumbs and wrist wraps, where less penetration is required. They are also available for backs and knees, but for these deeper areas I would strongly advise the use of neodymiums. A flexible magnet generally holds its field for 5–6 years.

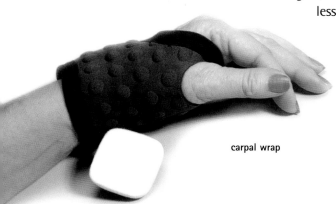

carpal wrap

As in the case of neodymiums – the surface area of contact with the body plays a vital part in the effectiveness of the fields. Due to the large area that is covered – flexible magnets can have a dramatic impact in the case of magnetic innersole/shoe inserts. Make sure the energy field of magnetic innersoles is throughout the sole. The fields will then 'hit' every reflexology point in the foot to maximise benefits.

CERAMIC MAGNETS

Ceramic magnets are generally found in pillow pads and sleep systems. You should look for ones with a gauss factor of over 3000 to promote relaxation whilst you sleep. They also kick in the pineal gland (remember Cleopatra!). Ceramic magnets are far less costly than neodymium, and so manufacturers can readily build them into large items, such as mattress pads at a fraction of the cost that neodymiums would be.

Most of the above magnets will be located with the NORTH POLE of the magnet towards the body. It is the general consensus that North Pole – heals, South Pole – stimulates. For healing, most companies use North Pole towards the body. Occasionally my therapists will treat a patient in their clinics with a limited exposure to South Pole, but the general rule I would recommend for you is to use North Pole magnets only. That is the general rule – of course there are always exceptions

INNERSOLES

are usually used by patients and athletes who are looking to improve circulation, energy and strength. They are also used for foot, ankle and lower leg pain.

Innersoles are usually BI-POLAR and FLEXIBLE. They will probably be sold in two or three sizes (small, medium and large). The customer will simply cut them down to size with a good pair of scissors. Magnetic soles will not take that much room in your shoes, and the results are certainly worth it.

powerstride – innersoles

WRISTBANDS AND BRACELETS

There are so many varieties of these particular magnetic devices now hitting the market and they are certainly worth looking at. Some are very pretty, but hardly effective, some are pretty ugly but powerful. The question you must ask yourself before you buy is:

"What do I want the bracelet to do for me?"

If your answer to the above question is for pain relief in the hand or wrist or for your general health and to help in your body's detoxifying process, then yes - buy a good wristband and keep it on. It is a simple and effective way of doing these things and it requires little effort. I wear a quality bracelet continuously, as do my therapists.

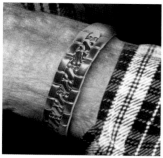

bracelet

Once again, insist on knowing the Gauss, surface and core, and get it in writing. Be sure of your supplier. A magnet of less than 800 GAUSS on the surface of your skin will give hardly any benefit. The one I wear has eight small neodymium magnets inset in a stainless steel link bracelet. The surface strength of each neo is 1,200 gauss. It is attractive, strong and powerful.

If your answer to the above question is that you want the bracelet for pain relief in your knee, forget it, (remember the lengthening and relaxing of tissue in the area!) As I said with directly applied high-grade magnets I would expect to see pain relief within hours or days.

Many bracelet companies will give you a 90 day money back guarantee, I presume this is because they think it will take that amount of time for the blood to circulate, cleanse the system of toxins and in so doing have an effect in the injured area. As a practising therapist I would not treat an injured area hoping a bracelet may eventually reach the site of injury. I would treat the site by direct application of the required magnets.

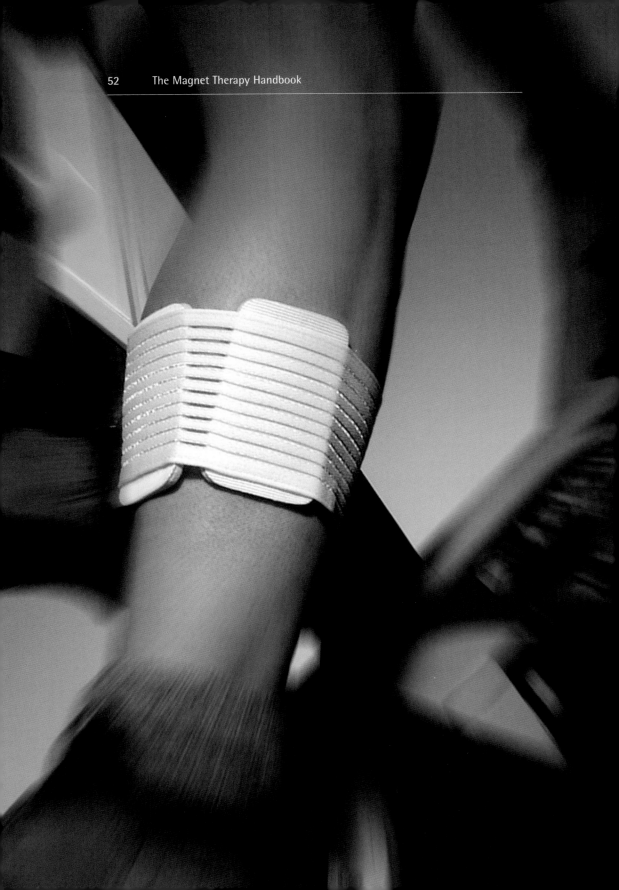

In conclusion

Apply the magnet to the site of your pain, and don't -"take a quarter of an aspirin for a headache – take the whole thing". Buy a quality product.

If you have absorbed most of the above information you will now know how to determine this. The rest is pretty easy. Most good manufacturers will have done the work for you. They understand when building their wraps e.g. for the knee, the penetration may have to reach 5-6 inches into tissue. So they will make the wrap with sufficient strength to do so. Manufacturers will not over build a product, so you may be sure they are safe for you to use freely as and when you want to.

When treating your family, be sure you have a complete understanding of what the trouble is, either by a diagnosis from your doctor or your specialist.

Even though there are no contra-indications and or 'side-effects' with magnet therapy we advise that the nature of the complaint be known i.e. If you have a pain in your chest – make sure your heart is OK! If you fall downstairs – make sure there are no broken bones!
Simple basic precautions for your sake.

TRAVEL AND MAGNET THERAPY

I love magnet therapy so much for two main reasons:

Once you buy them, YOU own them, and they work for you and your family, for years.

The other reason is that they are portable – they travel! Through airports, and they hold their field in all temperatures, cold, damp, humid or hot. They do not pass their 'sell by date!'

Sue Stockdale the first British
woman to walk to the North Pole

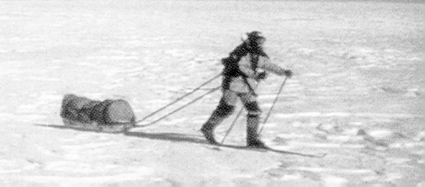

I have recently had the joy of providing two intrepid British Explorers (yes, they do still exist) with all sorts of goodies to take with them on their quests:

Sue Stockdale

My first challenge was a very plucky young woman named Sue Stockdale. Sue was the first British woman to walk to the North Pole (very appropriate for me!) I offered to supply Sue with magnetic innersoles to keep her feet warm and help restore and repair her energy over the gruelling trek she was undertaking across Greenland. She said thanks, but asked if there was any way we could make her a lightweight magnetic sleeping bag. This was an interesting project as Sue could not afford to carry too much excess weight other than supplies and clothing on her sled – but in turn, we needed to ensure enough magnetic field to give her sufficient overnight repair. Our research team in the USA came up with one, weighing under 2 kilos but with the power we felt she would need.

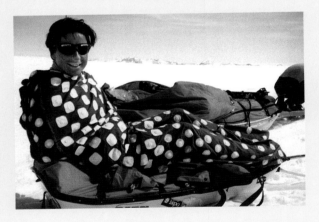

And here is a very contented Sue in the middle of the freezing snow and ice – looking her usual chirpy self. She wrote us a full and concise report on the usefulness and effectiveness of the sleeping bag and we learnt a lot from her comments.

"Thank you Norstar, your sleeping bag was the best piece of equipment I took with me.

I could count on it to keep me warm and offer me a really sound sleep, but best of all I was up and raring to go in the morning with no stiffness or achy limbs."

Colonel Blashford-Snell OBE

I first met the Colonel as he was about to leave on a trip to South America. He was returning to visit a tribe of isolated Indians in the heart of the Amazon rainforest, the reason – he had promised to take a grand piano (yes, I did say a grand piano) up the river, through the swamps and the rainforest and deliver it safely to the Wei -Wei tribe, who evidently lusted after one. I asked why they couldn't take a keyboard, but NO they wanted a grand piano, and the Colonel had promised them!

The Wei-Wei had recently converted to Christianity and they wanted their Sunday services to be accompanied by a grand piano! So naturally being the quintessential British Adventurer, the Colonel agreed to return with one.

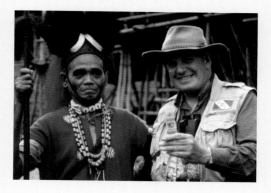

As the tribe had very little basic comforts and medicines were a luxury I agreed to provide the expedition with a selection of magnetic products.

It was then I found out that John had suffered for several years with very bad lower back problems. We gave him a lower back wrap and he was on the phone within hours of putting it on, raving about its success. Both he, and his wife have used our magnets for years now. (So presumably have the Wei-Wei)

> "I always carry the pad you gave me on all my expeditions and have used it on most parts of my body. I felt my back improving within hours. I now need a knee wrap for my wife."

Towards the end of this book you will find a section of treatment methods, this has been compiled to give you the general pointers you will need to use magnet therapy successfully.

SLEEP AND MAGNET THERAPY

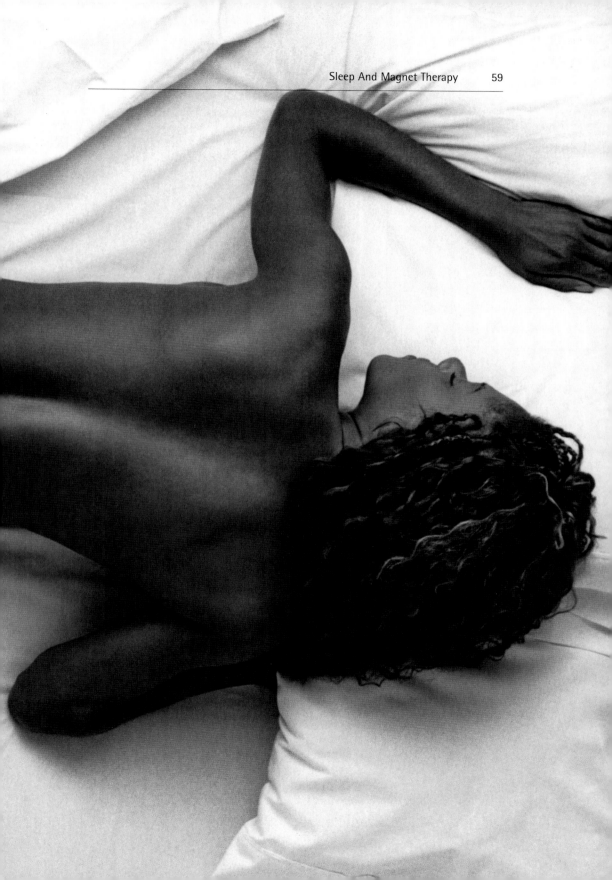

SLEEP AND MAGNET THERAPY

Just why are magnetic mattress pads such an incredible investment for your future health?

They are so because unlike 'spot' magnets the mattress pad bathes EVERY MUSCLE, CELL AND ORGAN in your body with a gentle magnetic field that is safe, natural and ESSENTIAL to our well-being. A good one will last 15 – 20 years and they require very little effort to use them.

Why do I think so highly of them? For several reasons...

Over 30% of the population does not get adequate sleep

Most of us are not really too sure what happens when we sleep, or what happens when we don't sleep. We do know that we would give a lot to be able to live our lives knowing we were going to get a good night's deep sleep and wake naturally, refreshed, relaxed and ready to go in the morning, every night for the rest of our lives. Just take a moment to think how that would affect you. Now read on to learn just how important sleep really is and just what does happen when we are deprived of it, and the simple solution to this problem, and many others.

What is sleep? Why do we need it?

Most people know that sleep provides physical rest; dreaming provides the mental equivalent of a cross-referencing and filing system. Some believe that the soul goes to a spiritual school, which we interpret as dreams. Whatever it is, we know that it is very important. Let's look at what else goes on while we sleep:

● Repair: some enzymes will switch on protein production for physical repair functions. Some cytokines will reinforce pathways in the brain to help memory and general functioning of the brain. We all know how our brains perform after a bad night! Other cytokines are important in empowering immune responses against illnesses including cancer.

● blood carries nutrients and oxygen around the system while it is relaxed and receptive

● Cleaning: the lymph system picks up waste from the cells and activates the immune system.

All these activities can be so easily compromised if the cells fail to receive the correct nutrients or if there is insufficient lymph/liquid/water to wash the system clean. Even worse is the fact that if we don't sleep sufficiently well for all this activity to be triggered off, it won't matter how good our diet or how much water we drink or how much we exercise, we will simply be losing out and getting older and sicker at a faster rate than is necessary.

Major problems associated with sleep deprivation

Most people know what it feels like to have had a bad night's sleep, but are you aware of just how badly it can affect your system?

- 3 hours sleep loss equates to a 50% reduction in our immune system activity

- Total sleep deprivation kills rats. On autopsy there is nothing wrong with them, they are actually killed by bacterial infections of the blood because their immune systems have crashed.

- Melatonin, secreted by the pineal gland, reaches its maximum about an hour after we fall into deep sleep. Only then do the body's repair functions respond and go into full swing.

Add to that a potentially harmful environment

The human body has developed over thousands of years to operate with and in the Earth's magnetic field. Magnetic energy is just one of the energy inputs our system needs. But now two things are happening simultaneously. First, the Earth's magnetic field is dropping significantly. NASA reports that it is as much as 14% down over the last 200 years and some respected scientists say it will go to zero before it starts to climb again. Secondly, the electro-magnetic environment we live in is being utterly corrupted by electric wiring, electric blankets, televisions and computers, mobile phones, etc. Even the US Surgeon General has warned of the harmful effects of this "electro-magnetic smog". A recent US report states that simply living in a concrete structure with iron and steel girders can insulate us from 50% of the natural geomagnetic fields we should be receiving.

How do magnets play their part?

Japan

Dr Shimodaira conducted a double-blind study of the effects of sleeping with a magnetic mattress pad across three hospitals in Tokyo.

Of the 375 subjects who slept on "real" magnetic pads:

- 301 (80.27%) reported positive results.

- 74 cases (19.73%) reported no results and not one person reported any side effects.

- 53% could tell the difference within 3 days, 70% within 5 days.

Dr Shimodaira's conclusion of the yearlong study conducted in 3 of Japan's foremost hospitals noted the following.
"The magnetised health mattress (pad) has proved to be effective on neck and shoulder pain, back and lower back pain, general back pain, lower limb pain, insomnia and fatigue, and to have no side effects."
American Health Magnetics, 1997

Europe/US

Realising the importance of sleep the Biotonus Clinique Bon Poert, one of Europe's best-known longevity clinics, uses Symtonic therapy to treat sleep disorders. This consists of a small silver device that is placed on the tongue for 20 minutes every evening. It emits electro-magnetic pulses! This has also been tested in the US where they noticed patients usually reduced the time taken to fall asleep by 45 minutes and increased the length of time for which they slept by 2 hours, all with no intolerance, rebound or adverse side-effects.

CASE STUDIES

General insomnia

At 62 John was getting up tired every morning after eleven hours sleep and couldn't drive for more than 30 minutes without falling asleep at the wheel. Since acquiring his magnetic mattress pad he sleeps better for less hours and recently drove 400 miles with no problems!

Shoulders and neck plus general stiffness

Jennifer, a top corporate executive at 50, was very frightened that she was becoming an old woman at 52. She had continuous pain in neck and shoulders and weakness in her arms. Walking upstairs became difficult and getting up in the morning took forever as she got her joints working after the stiffening up overnight. A friend suggested a magnetic mattress pad. Very sceptically she agreed to try one for a few nights. After just 2 nights she bought the pad from her friend!

Accident agony

By the time he was 35 David was in serious trouble. He had been an exceptional athlete, but the twice-broken leg and the dislocated shoulder were beginning to be painful and parts of his spine were starting to deteriorate. He was in permanent discomfort, at the very least, 24 hours a day. Then he had a car accident. One doctor suggested a morphine pump, another, further surgery. A friend recommended while making up his mind he should try a 5" x 7" magnetic pad. It was brilliant! He obtained some more magnetic devices and finally a magnetic mattress pad. He now sleeps all night with no pain and has fewer problems during the day. "I have no idea how it works, but it does."

Conclusion

Noticing something, studying it and then describing it such that predictions may be made of its behaviour defines true science. Just because detailed descriptions do not exist of how something functions doesn't mean it doesn't function, it just means the scientists have still got more work to do. We may not understand how electricity and magnetism function, but you don't stop to ask how does the TV work before you watch the weekly football match!

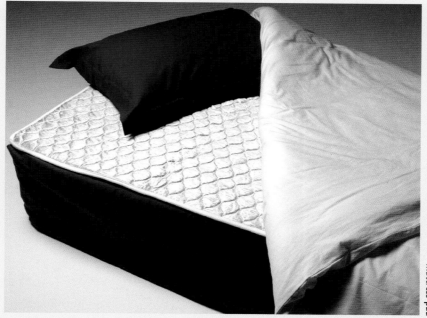

mattress pad

You know which switch, which channel and what time, all gleaned from other people, listings and your own personal experience. It's the same with magnetic mattress pads. The anecdotal information is extensive, the scientific studies have been done and have shown the product to be successful. The only possible adverse effect is that it will be bad for business for pharmaceutical companies who won't be selling you as many pills for the rest of your life!

Magnetic mattress pads work! They require no effort on your part, simply go to bed, get a good night's rest and wake feeling relaxed and ready to go!

MAGNETS IN SPORT

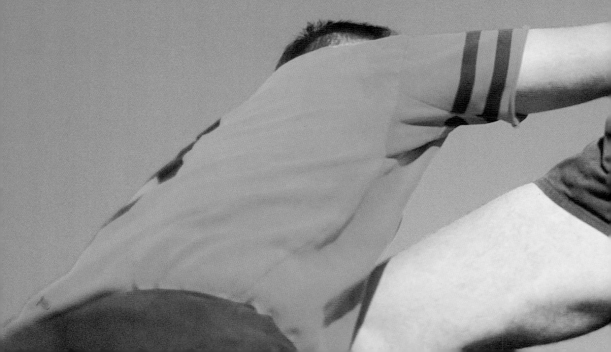

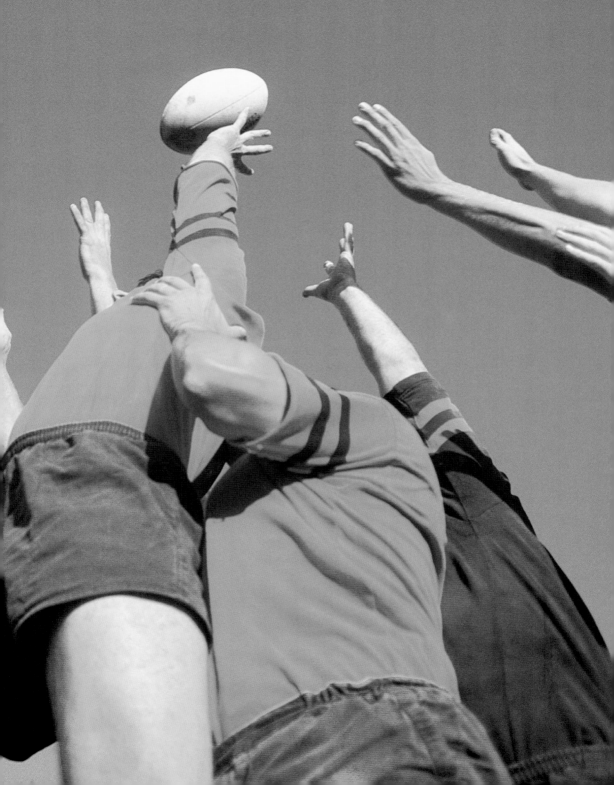

MAGNETS IN SPORT

ITS HERE TO STAY AND ITS LEGAL

Magnets involve no illegal chemicals that can contaminate blood or urine testing. As far as Olympic regulations go – they are no different to hot water bottles.

Earlier this year when I was attending a conference with the British Football Association, I had a chance to have a conversation with one of the medical advisors from FIFA (the controlling body for international soccer). The conclusion was once again, they could see no reason why these modalities could not be used legally in sport medicine.

Jack Scott, a member of the medical staff for the Summer Olympic Games, says he has seen so many athletes restored to competitive condition with magnets:

"The relief from pain associated with conditions such as chronic lower back pain, tendonitis, hamstring pulls, jumper's knee and muscular inflammation has made me a great believer."
Jack Scott

There is no longer any doubt about the effectiveness of magnets in sport. The list is endless and the results are now so impressive that it is an established addition to the medical bags and rehab equipment that follow the pro players around the circuits.

I will now list just a few of top athletes who now sing the praises of magnet therapy and are on record endorsing its value. This is not just to name-drop and impress you, it is to indicate both the recognition this means of pain control and rehabilitation is attracting, and more importantly, the fact that it is safe and it works. Not one of the managers or doctors of these 'multi-million dollar bodies' would risk them to a slightly wacky or dubious therapy.

Sport

It is estimated that well over 70% of all Senior PGA Golfers regularly wear magnets, including Arnold Palmer, Jim Colbert and Bob Murphy
Jim Colbert had been crippled since his youth with terrible pain in his back, and to quote Jim, "I haven't missed a day of golf in three years. Now I can swing just as well on the last hole as I do on the first. I couldn't play without using magnets. I guarantee you. Now I just play with two coin sized magnets (Neo's) strapped to my back."
So do Donna Andrews, Chi Chi Roderiguez and John Houston, who have both all gone on to buy full mattress pads.

In Tennis, Linzi Davenport had stopped playing about four years ago due to tennis elbow, she had been having intense physio for six months then a friend recommended magnets. As she said, she never looked back from that time. Whenever she over extends the arm, she re-applies the magnets. The same goes for both Jimmy Connors (knees) and John McEnroe (general aches and strains).

In Skiing, Mark Absalom was almost prohibited from competing by chondromalacia, arthritic knee. He used the Neo and a mattress pad, and then threw away his pain killers.

US Football – Bill Romanowski, who enjoys his reputation as the meanest linebacker in pro football (the Broncos), credits magnets for getting him pain-free, off anti-inflammatories and back on the team.

"I know what a great difference magnets have made to my life. I would like to help anyone else I can, feel this great."   Dan Marino Miami Dolphins.

CASE STUDY

**World Cup Mountain Biker
Will Corry Jnr**

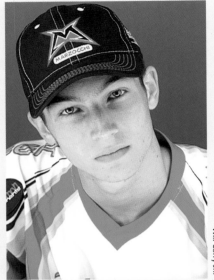

Will Corry Jnr

Will found out last year just how effective magnets can be. He is one a of those crazy guys who hurl themselves down mountains, over tree roots, bumps and pits every weekend for the hell of it.

I had done quite a lot of work with the cycle industry in the UK, and they have proved to be a really receptive group in trying and testing out magnet therapy. We can help prevent quite a lot of the jarring and bruising that is so common in their sport.

Will had heard about us on the grapevine and contacted us after he broke his scaphoid in his wrist, following a heavy fall in a World Cup downhill event in Durango, Colorado. He was also badly bruised in several places. We sent him a magnetic massage machine, and several wraps and disks to use on the various damaged parts of his body. We also included a mattress pad as part of his recovery programme. I am pleased to say that Will was back competing within weeks. His coach was so amazed and delighted with the

simplicity of magnets, and the fact that they could self-treat, following a simple conversation with us. That he and his team mates now carry around a full kit bag of various products to wrap and strap every part that gets continually beaten up.

The mattress pad is now shared out to the most needy member of the team.

Will Corry Jnr
IRELAND NATIONAL WORLD CUP TEAM RIDER

I will not bore you with endless lists, but as you can see most of the above athletes are from the USA where the explosion of magnet therapy is quite recent. In the UK, it is beginning the same way that it did in the USA, it is being driven by the general public, then by word of mouth they are involving their health care professionals and gradually we are making inroads and gaining acceptance with the relevant authorities, but WHY does it take so long here – just slap one on, and watch what happens – It is really that simple.

I regularly have both professional and general everyday riders using innersoles to great benefit.

Many top professional sportsmen are now using them either for repair, endurance or to enhance their performance.
The innersoles are terrific used in sports which 'traumatise' the feet.
Prime examples of these activities are running and kickboxing. The athlete will use the innersole in their shoes after the event in order to bring in the extra oxygen and blood flow to start repairing the area and flush out the lactic acid that has built up.

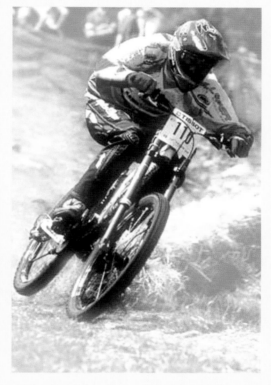

For events that use a shoe that can take the extra sole and who do not require the agility of a runner, typical examples are: skiing, skating, weight lifting, golf and tennis, then the magnetic innersole is worn to enhance the performance. I have been told that The British Federation of Ice Skating is currently trying to ban innersoles as an "unfair advantage".

Why? Just wear them as the rest of the world does!

CASE STUDY

Iron man, Tri–athlete Athlete/Journalist
Bill Davis

Two years ago a British tri-athlete sportsman came to me and asked if I could work with him to improve his performance.

He asked: "Could magnet therapy speed the recovery time from injuries he periodically received from the various disciplines (running, swimming and cycling) he competed in?"

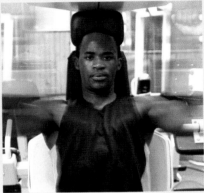

His nutrition and training regimes were fine so we looked in the areas of strength, energy and stamina.

We decided to use the following items:

The 'poker chip' neodymium disks. These small disks are the size and weight of a 2p coin. Our tri-athlete could keep them with him in his first aid kit and then place anywhere on his body should he pull or strain a muscle. They would alleviate the pain and speed the healing process. We also suggested that Bill should use them on his lower back when he cycled to off-set the normal ache he would get during the long cycling events.

A sleep system. He took a single mattress pad around with him to place on his bed at night.

I tease him that he is cheating. He tells me its ergogenics!

The mattress pad allowed him to get a deeper 'alpha' state of sleep, to recover from the exhaustion of the day's events and wake with increased energy and without the tired muscles.

Supreme Innersoles:

The innersoles were used after his running races, to repair the damage to the feet.

He used the innersoles during the cycling events to add power and stamina to the legs. After a 112-mile training session he reported that at the 92-mile point he just left his teammates behind. He knew that normally they were all pretty well matched. He re-tested them the following week and confirmed the extra performance the innersoles gave him. Bill now wears them for all his races.

I mentioned earlier, that many countries use them regularly. It is not new, or avant-garde, any longer, just normal practice. In the UK, we are only recently becoming aware of the benefits magnetic field therapy can bring

Awareness is growing

We now have calls daily from premier league soccer clubs, golfers, rowers, weight lifters, skaters, asking for advice and information.

'How to heal this fracture?'

'How to relax this torn muscle?'

'How to ease my back?'

The age of magnets in sport is here – ask the rest of the world!

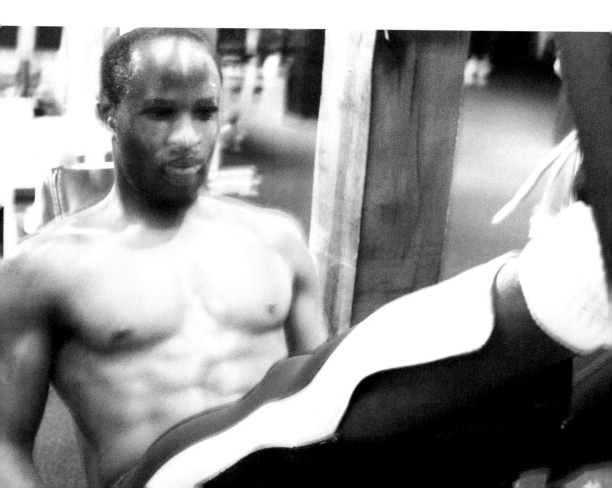

LET'S LOOK AT THE BEAUTY ASPECT

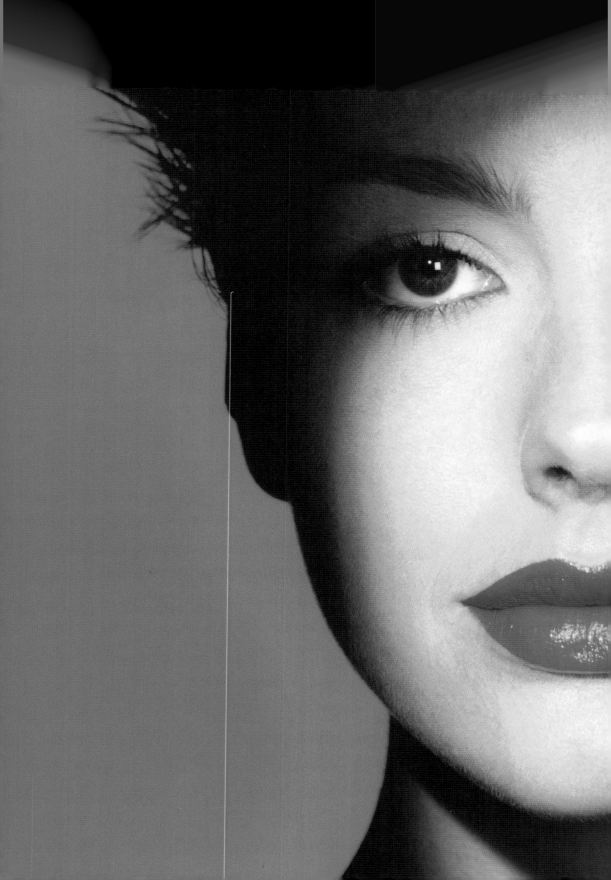

LET'S LOOK AT THE BEAUTY ASPECT

Almost side-effects in magnet therapy are the benefits and improvements it can bring to the skin, hair and nails. This is largely due to the increase in oxygen and blood flow magnets bring with them. It is almost the same 'rush' as doing an aerobic work out or, more specifically, having a great massage.

When you have a facial, and the beauty therapist is massaging your face, most of the work is in the stimulation of cells, renewed oxygenation and encouragement of the lymph system to give up some of the 'debris' that naturally clings to the walls of our cells. The specific creams used play only a part in that repair or 'beauty treatment' as we commonly call it.

The same activity occurs when magnets are used, namely increased blood flow and lymphatic drainage. We all know how wonderful a good massage feels, there is nothing quite like it. Touch is so sensual and indeed, essential, to our overall sense of feeling good. But, just consider having the luxury of an eight-hour facial massage every night. This is what happens when my patients use a magnetic pillow pad or sleep system. Very often our customers have bought the pad to ease stress and depression, or to promote sleep, but the side effects are so often a vibrant and radiant, glowing skin, brighter and less puffy eyes, glossy hair and better-conditioned nails.
Not bad for a side effect.

WATER   WATER   WATER!

"Is it that important?"
Yes, I promise you it is. Please drink a minimum of four glasses a day. Ideally the experts tell us to drink 2 litres. If you can manage that your body will love you for it. Personally as one who considered a drink during the day as tea or coffee, I am happy to do 3 - 4 glasses. In the winter try drinking it hot. I know it does not sound too good but I promise you, you will get use to it. And don't worry, it is tea and coffee that are the diuretics. Take it from the greatest bathroom seeker in the world, water helps to dilute the effects of caffeine. My daily regime is to have my morning cup of tea, followed by a decaffeinated coffee. From then on, I am on water. I may possibly have another tea or coffee during the afternoon but usually that's it. And, as one who looks forward to her G&T or glass of wine with dinner, I try to drink a glass of water at night once again to dilute the alcohol.

Get into the routine of drinking water; it's worth it. We know we are made up of over 75% water, what must happen to our cells if we deprive our bodies and dehydrate them? Just think what happens when we do not water our plants regularly - they droop and sag. Well, the same thing happens to us. We do not sag exactly because we have a skeletal structure holding us upright – but we droop nevertheless!

As a dancer I have grown up with the understanding that the body is our vehicle, the working, moving part 'of us'. It takes me from place to place - not the car. Think about it. It is our body that gets us to the car or bus. Without maintaining this incredible machine we are nowhere. It is the greatest piece of engineering I know of, nothing equals it and it is my aim to 'die fit'. To do that I will feed it with good stuff (whole foods), exercise it periodically, and WATER it.

The rest is up to my magnets.

Since I have been using magnet therapy, which is coming up to six years, I have not had a cough or cold, my immune system is in terrific shape and I can also speak for my therapists and friends who use it regularly.

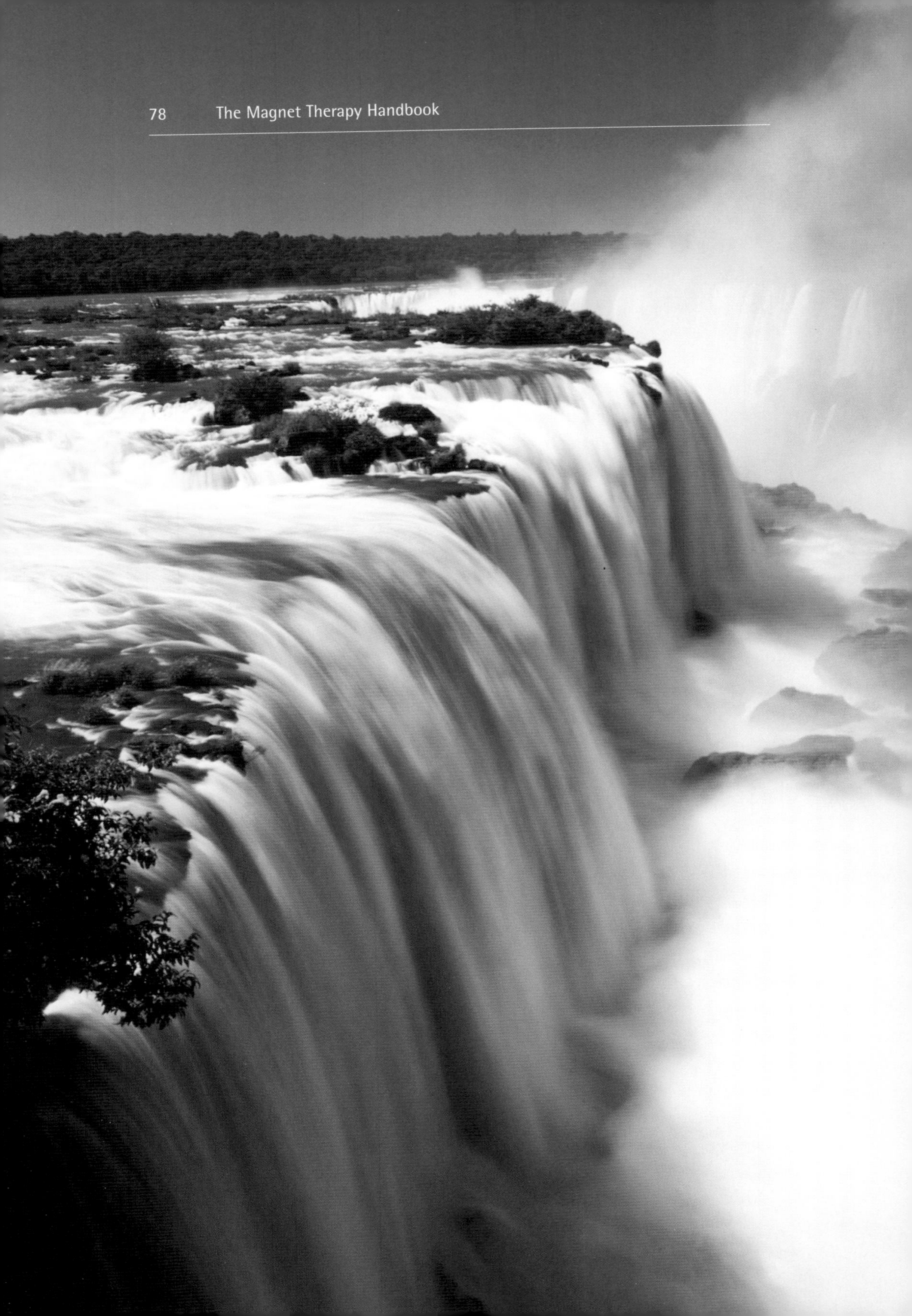

How to Magnetise Water

For many conditions, including colitis, eczema or psoriasis, we recommend drinking magnetised water.
For fuller details see the Treatment section on p.100

Any water can be magnetised; it is simple. Just place your jug or glass on a magnetic block or a specially designed Water Coaster for 20 minutes for a glass, and allow about 1 hour for a full bottle of or jug. The water will then hold the magnetic properties for days.

NORTH POLE WATER

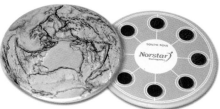

coaster

> Calming and Relaxing.
> Used for most conditions.
> Place the container on the block
> with the North Pole facing upwards.

SOUTH POLE WATER

> For Stimulation and Energy. Place the container on the block with the South Pole facing upwards.

BIPOLAR WATER

> For Balance and Harmony
> Place a South Pole magnet on one side of the container and a North Pole on the other.
> Alternatively mix the two above waters together.

Handy Tip: If you have tomatoes, strawberries or any fruit - that are not quite ripe enough, just place them on a South Pole magnet, we find it speeds up the ripening process.

A great tip I love!

> If you have a bottle of wine that is very rough and harsh to drink place the bottle on a magnetised water coaster or simply tape a Neodymium disk to the bottle with the North Pole towards the wine. Leave it there for about 30 minutes, then see how it smoothes the taste out, the wine should become fuller and sweeter to the palate. If you place the bottle on the South Pole - watch out - it will become more acidic.

FOR YOU AND YOUR PETS TOO

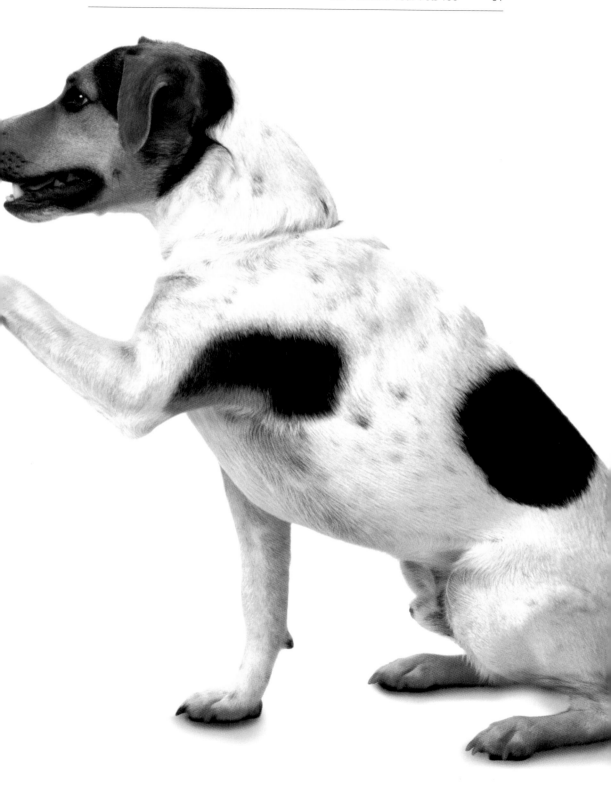

FOR YOU AND YOUR PETS TOO

One of the nicest things we find in magnet therapy is watching the difference we can make to our four legged friends. Getting positive results when dealing with animals is satisfying for two reasons...

...of course it is rewarding to help a cat, dog, rabbit or horse in pain, that goes without saying.

The real buzz comes from the knowledge that the animal is not expecting anything to happen. When a dog with an arthritic hip responds because its owner has put magnets in its bed or on its collar -well that's a different thing entirely. It reinforces our commitment every time. You will see some of our work with animals in the personal testimonials in a later chapter. In animals as with people we can help with arthritis, oedema (swelling) and faster recovery from damage or operations.

Following the initial studies into the use of magnetic fields, during the initial years of space exploration, the first group of outsiders who really took up the use of modern therapeutic magnets in a big way was the racing industry in the USA.

Used primarily on horses, blankets were made housing powerful magnets. These were positioned all over the cover so the animals could get the benefits whilst travelling to the meetings in their boxes and maintain them during their time in the parade ring. The effect was to calm down the more nervous horses, but more importantly to help 'warm up' the muscles and get them primed for their race.

The horse racing industry travels the world and for years they have been aware of the useful part magnet therapy can play in their sport. You can find wraps for fetlocks, hooves and shins, and blankets, that help with the warm up process before a race. Again the magnetic wand (magnessage) is a great tool to use with horses. On several occasions I have worked with animals that were skittish and difficult to shoe. We found that passing the wand around the head for a minute or two, the horses would then calmly give their hoof to the blacksmith.

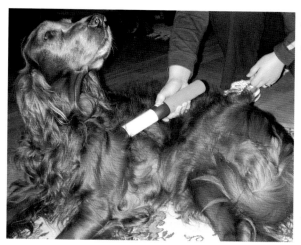

Magnessage

One little story I must tell you happened two years ago as I was coming home from a talk I was giving on Magnet Therapy. I was returning from Shepton Mallet on my way to Bath when I noticed a group of people surrounding an animal at the side of the road. I could see the little creature was in spasm, so I grabbed my Magnessage and over I went. It turned out to be a small deer that had been hit by a car. The crowd had covered its head, to not shock it further, and two men were holding its legs. Without touching the deer I passed the Magnessage over it (the field of penetration on this is 15 -18 inches) for a minute or so and the deer relaxed and stopped jerking. I then switched the Magnessage off and within 30 seconds the little thing was back jerking, again I began treatment again and she calmed down. I then carried on treating her until the RSPCA came. Unfortunately, her back was broken and she was put down. But what proof for me, that even with a wild animal who had her head covered, something tangible happened and something pretty significant. The onlookers were amazed to see what was happening and I had four customers before I got off my knees!

Time and time again my therapists and I see the healing in the horses and domestic animals we work with. I have recently been asked to work with a tiger in a local zoo. NOT my usual client, but I will have a go making sure there is qualified supervision standing by, else my ambition to 'die fit' may just come true a little ahead of schedule.

Once the word (and understanding) of the 'serious' side of this industry, gets out magnets will be on offer everywhere. Hopefully you will now be ahead of the game and know what to look out for and what to stay clear of.

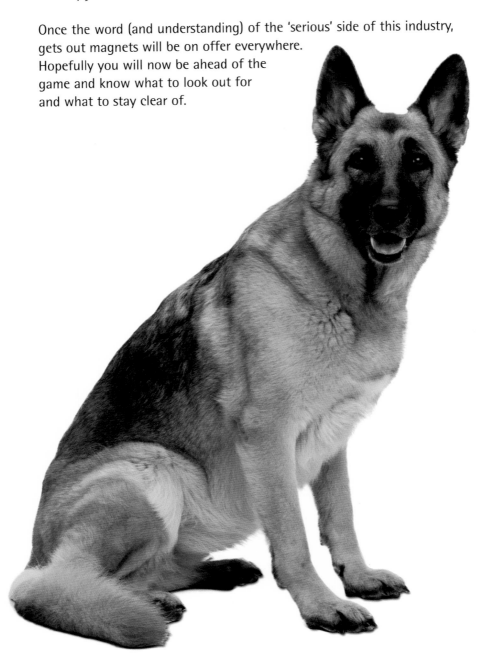

CASE STUDIES

Dear Gloria

I am writing to tell you about the Pet Pad (Pillow Pad) results seen in my German Shepherd. Chessie has hip dysplasia, and I think it took her less than a month to realise that the more time she spent on her pad the better she felt. In recent weeks I have started treating her with one of my Neo disks for a pulled tendon in her hind leg. She did the damage six months ago and showed no signs of recovering from it, despite the vet's help.

Within 24 hours of plastering a Neo inside her thigh, the limp became less pronounced and after 72 hours she walked without a limp. She is now bounding in and out of the car, and actually appears to be so much happier. Can you now send me out another set of Neos - in case I need them for my old hip trouble, I think I will treat myself to a Pillow Pad too!

Yours sincerely,
Anebell

SNAKES ALIVE!

One last little anecdotal story I have to mention happened when I was doing a two hour inter-active show I have on a TV channel in England. A caller rang to say what incredible results she had had in days, by sleeping on her mattress pad. Sandra was suffering from a serious immune deficiency problem and she just called to say 'thank you'. We chatted for a while and then she told me how much her pet corn snake....was also enjoying the pad. She told me how he kept disappearing all day to creep up on it, and absolutely 'insisted' on sleeping between her and her husband at night.

Well would you argue with a fully grown snake?

Seriously though – there is logic behind the snakes attraction to the mattress pad. Snakes naturally spend their lifetime outside, lying flat out with the entire length of their body on the earth. They, more than any other animal, should soak up all the magnetic fields their bodies can accept. I expect this little 'house snake' was somewhat deprived and sensed exactly where he should be!

IN CONCLUSION
WHERE IS IT GOING?

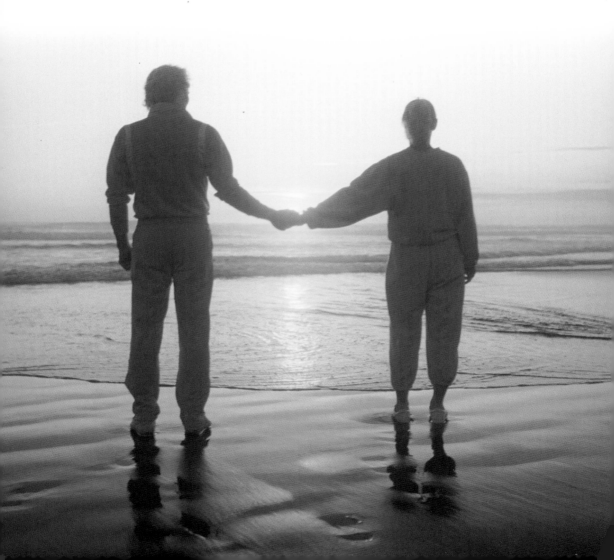

It is my honest belief that magnet therapy will be part of the NHS and UK medicine within five years. Its part in relieving pain and reducing symptoms in many of the areas I have described in this book are too vital to be ignored. By applying good quality magnets to people in industries where R.S.I (repetitive stress injury) is common, magnet therapy can very often offset the conditions arising, saving millions in lost man hours. Hopefully, we are now entering a new era where the medical profession will begin to take a long and hard look at the new science of 'energy medicine'. This will include vibrational sound and light therapies as well as several other forms, including magnetic field therapy, that are rapidly emerging.

The Chinese have taken energy fields seriously for centuries, and the Russians have done so since the sixties. Even with the resistance put up by the drug companies and the FDA, the American public have turned to it in their millions. Yes, millions.

According to Jim Souder, the founder of Norso Biomagnetics in the USA, "The modern magnets we use today are just the harbinger of where this technology will lead." From their clinics in the USA Drs Rosch and Lawrence have written, "Although one would have to say magnet therapy is still in the formative stage, its future looks bright with promise – very bright indeed. One might even add that, as we are naturally attracted to healing and relief from pain, magnet therapy is pulling us irresistibly towards forward."

So, as I mentioned earlier, know and understand the condition you want to treat. Feel free to share this book with your doctor or consultant. Most accredited therapists will be glad to answer any questions you may have. Further reading on this subject appears in the reference section of this book, together with some useful contact numbers.

For the sceptics out there I would say – you have nothing to lose, try it. Remember the old saying: "If it ain't broke, don't fix it." All of us in magnet therapy would like to say: "If it works, don't knock it."

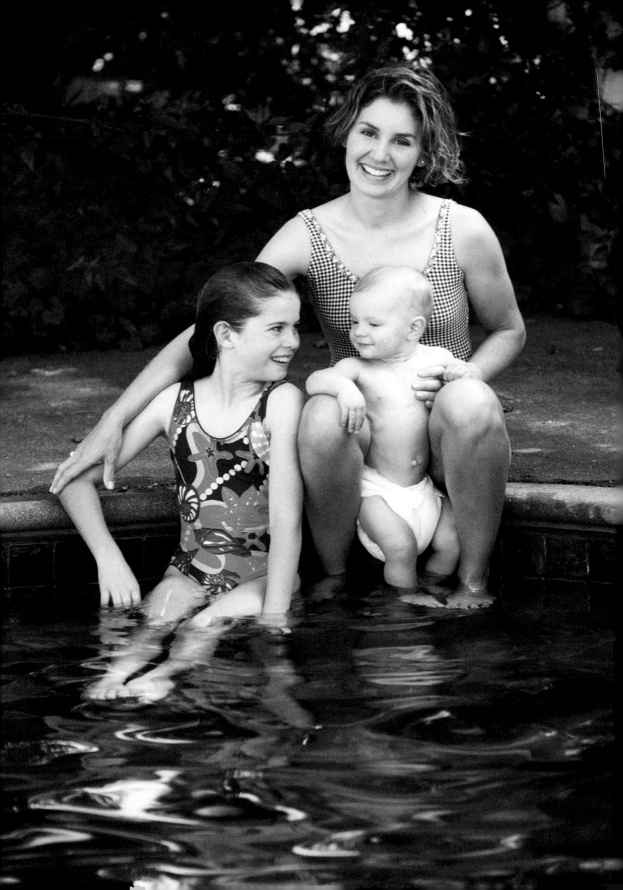

TESTIMONIALS

The following testimonials come from a few of the patients I have worked with and some from the casebooks of my therapists.
They are spontaneous and not solicited in any way.

Arthritis

Dear Gloria,

Thank you so much for all your help. I want you to have in writing how much your poker chips have helped my hip. They have also made the world of difference to my 9-year-old dog, Toby. Toby had been unable to walk with arthritis so for three weeks we have been sharing them! We are now both bounding with ease, but I feel I need my own set. Please send me another pair ASAP.

Sincerely, Julia Paton, Dernia Spain

To whom it may concern

As a concert pianist, my hands are vital to me. My arthritis was causing me so much pain I was in fear of not being able to perform. Your Neos, together with the Magnessage, have proved so successful that I have been granted a new lease on life, or certainly performing. Many thanks,

Sue Ross, Finchley London

Dear Gloria

After five years on painkillers – I am off them. I have had my first pain-free weekend and have been so ever since using Biomagnets. Thank you Gloria for coming to Bath.

Very sincerely,

Monica Brown, Bathwick, Bath

Blood Pressure

The benefits I have had since wearing my Link Bracelet are brilliant, my blood pressure has stabilised for the first time in a year and I am getting feeling back in my left foot which has had no feeling in it for about ten years since I slipped a disk. Many thanks,

Jan, email via Ideal World Shopping Channel

Carpal Tunnel & R.S.I.

Thank you so much for the magnetic link bracelet, I cannot understand how something so small can change my life and get me back to work in a day. My wrist has been an increasing problem for me over the past few years and the pain-killers were no longer working. This is a wonderful thing you have shown me.

Phillipe Dreux, Belpech, France

As you know I was very sceptical that magnets would help the R.S.I. / Arthritis I had suffered from for many years due to riding my motor bike and using the throttle.
But after wearing it overnight the pain in my thumb was gone. I was so impressed I lent it to my mother, she was so impressed she will not give it back.   Please send me another one. Thanks again.

Byron Lewis   Lower Weare, Somerset 1998

Fibromyalgia

The following three testimonials are from:
Christine Craggs-Hinton: Author "Living with Fibromyalgia"

'Gloria, I have to say I am staggered by how effective the magnets are! During the last few days I have been in less pain and have had far more energy than at any other time in the last eight years – and done things I thought I had lost forever, like driving a car. I feel like I am getting my life back, which is absolutely brilliant!'
Shipley May 28th 2000

'I'm back after a great holiday! The sunshine did me a lot of good. I took my mattress pad with me which kept my usual problem of 'holiday constipation' at bay, it also helped me stay more active than ever before since I became ill.
Shipley 18th July 2000

'Did I mention my mattress pad has completely stabilised my IBS (irritable bowel syndrome) – which as you know often comes with Fibromyalgia?'
Shipley 26th July 2000

Lymphoedema

Dear Gloria

Shortly after wearing my magnets I noticed a marked reduction in the pain I had had from lymphoedema following a radical mastectomy for breast cancer five years ago. In due course the swelling in my arm subsided and is now, what is described as "within normal limits". Thank you so much, and also thanks for the follow up calls and advice.

Marian Jackson, Bournemouth

(referred to us by the Royal Bournemouth Hospital, Breast Care Dept.)

Gloria,

You have changed my life. After using your poker chips I have got my life back. I am a nearly new person. My lymphoedema is now controlled and the pillow pad has helped with sleep and stress. My friends are all shocked and so happy for me. Thanks for being there.

Sandra Rose, Poole Dorset.

(also from the Royal Bournemouth Hospital, Breast Care Dept)

CASE STUDY

Spinal Muscular Atrophy

Judi Wolfenden
Following The London to Jerusalem Endurance Car Rally.

I have had the privilege to know Judi for a few years and she is inexhaustible. Judi has spinal muscular atrophy, but you would never know it. She hang glides, bunji jumps – you name it and if it is for a good cause, she will try it. I have been amazed by Judi's determination on a number of occasions especially when she connives to get me involved in some of her events – such as the Flora London Women's Challenge 2000. Both of us being the competitive souls we are – we were the first wheel chair entries past the finish line. Nice one!
Judi now wants me to do the New York Marathon ...NOT so nice!!

"I was naturally apprehensive about taking part in the rally, so each morning I put on the back wrap, and to my amazement was completely free of pain. In fact the only time on the rally that I had any intense pain was during the ceremony at the Besor Reservoir,

when a professional photographer (laden with camera equipment) slipped and fell on top of me.

"Thank you for generously giving me the Norstar wraps, this special item ensured that I was free of pain."

Judi now plans to do the next one on a Harley !!

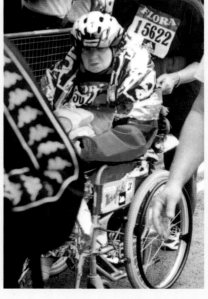

Flora London Women's Challenge 2000.

Stress & Depression

I have only been on the mattress pad for three nights and already I can feel the difference. It is beginning to ferry me around and help me out of the deepest troughs both mentally and physically. Please call as I want to discuss another of your products for a friend and my mother.

Claire Calascione, Bristol

Dear Gloria
Thank you for sending me the pillow pad so quickly. I already feel so different wearing the innersoles.
I now feel my breakdown is far behind me, maybe I am at last producing my own serotonin. I think you have changed my life irreversibly for the better. I cannot thank you enough!
I allowed my daughter to wear them for her SATS yesterday!
It was lovely to meet you.

Annabel Jones Lancashire, May 2001

Tendon and Muscle Pain

To you all,
I wish I could truly express how I feel since I started your magnets. The discomfort and pain I have felt for years has disappeared. I also believe the support and help I received from you on the phone was of such benefit I have been singing your praises ever since.
Many thanks, sincerely

Betty Talbot, Walton-on Thames

Tel message:

"Gloria, I just called to say thank you for the little disks. They are tremendous. As you may remember I am a professional guitarist. My R.S.I. was interfering with my playing and I was terribly worried. Now, as soon as I feel any strain coming in my hand I tape the disks on and – problem solved. I have learnt to put them on if I know I have a heavy session coming up and I do not set up the pain. It has made such a difference to my me and my career. Thanks, a pal of mine will be calling you shortly.

Richard, Bath, Avon 1999

Tennis Elbow

I am writing to say that I am a complete convert to magnet therapy. I was getting a lot of pain from my neck down to my elbow, and was unable to use that arm. I ordered a Link Bracelet and the pain went completely. When I returned to my chiropractor he said that the inflammation was gone from the site and that magnets were allowing my body to heal, as it should. I tell everyone that will listen about magnets. Thank you so much for your help and advice.

Valerie, email via Ideal Shopping Channel

Making it all Worthwhile

Following is a completely unsolicited letter from a customer, James Astley. The Astley family have since become very precious to everyone in our office, and we all wish Rhiannon year and years of good health.

A brief history:

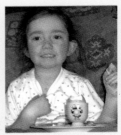

Rhiannon Astley

Rhiannon Astley – 3 years of age, born with a hole in her heart, which was also reversed. When James first called us, we naturally asked for some background on Rhiannon. Once we understood a little about her condition we realised how we could help. Due to her young age we wanted to work slowly, and give her time to adjust easily to the increased oxygen flow. During the initial few days, her parents carefully monitored her response. We had asked James to place a large pillow pad in Rhinnaon's bed. Instead of placing it directly under her chest area, we told James to place it under her bottom for a few days to let her body become used to the effects of added fields and then after a few days, he gradually eased the pad up so it was under her upper body.

Dear Gloria

Thank you for the get well card for my daughter Rhiannon. Because of her condition she had very poor oxygen saturation, after speaking to you we decided to get a stress buster for her to sleep and sit on. The effects were almost immediate, her colour improved and she slept better; she also had more energy throughout the day. From a little girl with no energy, within days she was chasing her cousins around the house.

As you know she had her open heart surgery a lot sooner than we had expected. Rhiannon suffered from transposition of the great arteries, with a ventricular septal defect and a pulmonary stenosis. This means her heart is the wrong way round with a hole between the pumping chambers and a very small pulmonary valve

Her surgery began at nine o'clock on the 25th of July (2002) and was supposed to last for eight hours but after five hours we received a pager message to phone the surgeon. Fearing the worst we rang only to be told the team had finished and everything went very well. Then at four o'clock we were allowed to see her on ICU. She looked great even though she was still heavily sedated. At half past five the biggest shock came as she started to wake up and tried to remove the respirator tubes, which were at this time doing all the breathing for her. When the nurse asked her if the pipes were annoying her she started to nod, which surprised the nurse as she was still sedated. They took her off the machine and she began to breath on her own much to everyone's surprise. By seven o'clock she began demanding a drink. The following morning they removed the drain tubes from her chest and by one o'clock they took her back down to the ward. By the evening she was sitting up in bed asking me to bring in her favourite videos. They moved her from the high-care side of the ward, to the normal ward.

On Monday we saw the surgical team who were all astounded by her recovery, they said they had never seen a child recover so quickly from this type of corrective surgery, and we brought her home on Friday 2nd of August. We believe that the speed of her recovery was due to the magnet therapy as it must of boosted her immune system etc. Looking at her it is hard to believe that only a week ago she had major heart surgery, as the scar is now only a very thin red line. I am telling everybody I know about your products.

We would be honoured to have Rhiannon in your book and you don't have to change the name or area. I have said before, I would speak to anyone who has a child with a heart condition to assure them of the benefits of your products. We told several parents whilst we were at the hospital and all of them were very interested in the mattress covers so I told them to either go to your web site or to ring you for more information. We have also been talking to the cardiac liaison nurses, as they were interested as well. Alder Hey has a very large Oncology department so we will pass on your information to them. As soon as we can, we'll get them to ring you, but as you know hospital admin can move as slow as a dinosaur. Thank you for all your help.

James Astley

TREATMENTS 'HOW TO TREAT'

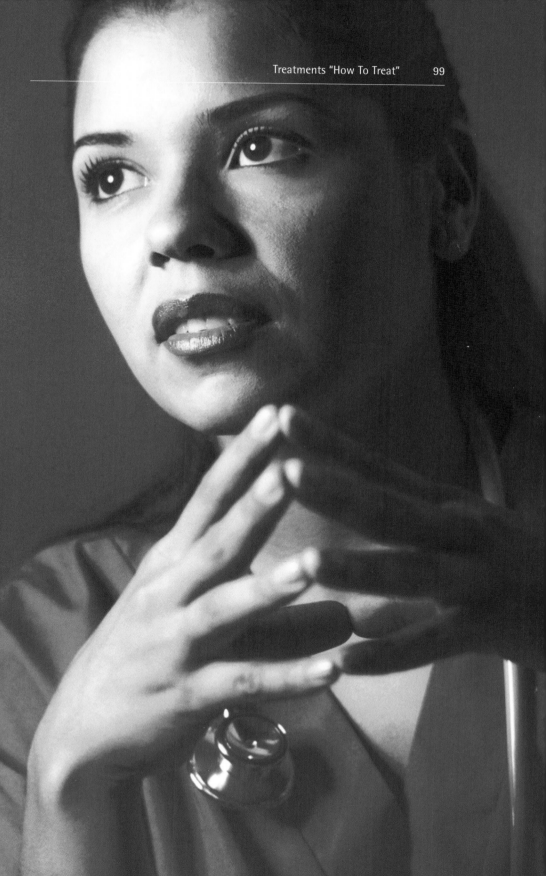

TREATMENTS 'HOW TO TREAT'

As I have said, the important fact that differentiates magnet therapy from other forms of treatments – is that you – or rather you and Nature together – become the 'healers'.

Most good magnet therapy practitioners are really consultants. They are there to understand the condition you have, judge your degree of pain, understand your mobility and lifestyle and then offer you perhaps a treatment or two - then to advise on the best product for your needs.

The glory of this method of healing is IT'S YOURS and it's yours for many years. I have gathered the following list from far and wide - from studies done in many of the world's top clinics and hospitals. I have only listed conditions where I believe significant benefits can be seen.

You will see I have recommended the use of (NORTH POLE) mattress pads for many conditions, if this is not affordable for you at the moment, try to buy a smaller type of magnetic sleep system such as a pillow pad or slightly larger product that is available in the market.

DO NOT USE MAGNET THERAPY IF YOU HAVE A PACEMAKER, DEFIBRILLATOR, INSULIN PUMP OR IF YOU ARE PREGNANT

Throughout this book I have emphasised the need to think just what you really want magnet therapy to do for you. I will briefly summarise what has gone before.

I have emphasised the importance of water throughout this book; I know many of us are not in the habit of picking up a glass of water, but please do so. Think of it as a vital part of your treatment. We want the toxins that will be released from your system to be effectively flushed out as waste. It is a good idea to start drinking water 2 - 3 days before you begin your treatment. Carry on drinking it – Forever forever

PAIN RELIEF IN SPECIFIC AREAS OF THE BODY

Apply the appropriate magnetic wrap or disk to the site. In some severe cases I suggest you keep the magnet in place for a few hours, give yourself a break of an hour then re apply. After your body has become accustomed to the magnet you are free to leave the wrap or disk in place for as long as you feel you need to.

Ongoing conditions:
The magnet can be used daily or nightly. If the major part of your pain is during the day wear the magnet then. If you can maintain the benefits simply by wearing it at night do so.

For example use Innersoles for:
ENERGY, CIRCULATION, FOOT AND LOWER LEG PAIN , TO ENHANCE YOUR PERFORMANCE IN SPORTS

THE A TO Z OF MAGNET THERAPY TREATMENTS

ACNE

Results in treating acne vary greatly from patient to patient, but I would certainly give magnet therapy a try. I suggest the following: Wear a magnetic bracelet on the left hand. Drink magnetised water and bathe the areas in magnetised water. Magnetise your creams by using the North Pole of a magnet (towards the cream). Use a magnetic mattress Pad.

ADRENAL GLANDS

Use magnetic innersoles. Use a magnetic mattress pad.
Drink North Pole magnetised water.

AGEING

Drink North Pole magnetised water. Use magnetic innersoles.
Use a magnetic mattress pad.
Use a Pillow Pad to boost oxygen enriched blood flow to the face.

ALLERGIES

Help to boost your immune system by using a bracelet and some form of sleep system for night repair.
Drink North Pole magnetised water.

AMPUTATION PAIN

We have had excellent results treating phantom leg pain by having patients sit on a pillow pad, or target treat the area with Neodymium disks.

neodymiun disc

ARTHRITIS

Our results in significantly relieving the discomfort and pain associated with arthritis are remarkable. Apply wraps or Neodymium disks directly over the affected part of the body, as and when it is required. If the arthritis is in several areas of the body, the use of a mattress pad is recommended. Use magnetic innersoles. Drink North Pole magnetised water.

ASTHMA

Wear a magnetic bracelet. Use a small pad or 1/2" Neo disks in the chest area.

BACKACHE

Use of a lower back wrap or 1 "Neodymium disks applied to the site. Use a magnetic mattress pad.

BITES AND STINGS

First, be sure the bite or sting is not poisonous – consult a doctor or pharmacist if you are not sure.
Clean and rinse the area with vinegar or another disinfectant, apply a 1/2" Neo to the area.

BLADDER PROBLEMS

Sitting on a magnetic pillow pad has proved to be beneficial in many cases if an infection is present. Try using a pad applied to the area. Drink North Pole magnetised water.

BLOOD PRESSURE – LOW

Wear a good quality magnetic bracelet on the Left Hand.

BLOOD PRESSURE – HIGH

Wear a good quality magnetic bracelet on the Right Hand. Work in conjunction with your doctor so results can be monitored, and see whether medication can be reduced.

BRONCHITIS

Apply a small magnetic pad or 1/2" Neos over the chest area. Keep in place for four hours the first day, and then increase its daily use as you judge the benefits require. Monitor your degree of comfort in using the pad. Sit on a pillow pad. Drink North Pole magnetised water.

BONES – BROKEN OR FRACTURED

Once you have had the bone or fracture 'set' use magnets to encourage the bone to knit. We regularly place 1" Neodymium magnets on the outside of a plaster cast. They will penetrate well into the cast and body to speed the healing.

BRUISING

For falls or severe bruising due to accidents – consult your doctor. On minor bumps and bruising – apply a North Pole Neodymium disk immediately to the site.

BURNS AND SCALDS

For severe burns and scalds consult your doctor.
For minor burns and scalds, bathe the affected part gently with cold water (North Pole magnetised if available) - apply a North Pole Neodymium disk immediately to the site.

BURSITIS

Use a wrap on the affected area.
Wear a good quality magnetic bracelet.

CANCER

Cancer of course is a major cause of concern and one of our biggest killers. Magnet therapy cannot claim any part in the treatment of the disease. All we can hope for is to relieve some of the associated discomfort and to encourage the immune system to recover and 'fight back' after the necessary treatments and drugs that are prescribed. I suggest you call our telephone helpline for advice; or one of the recommended therapists listed at the back of this book. General advice would be to wear a good quality magnetic bracelet and use some form of sleep system.
Drink North Pole Water.

CHRONIC FATIGUE SYNDROME

Move as many electrical appliances from the vicinity of your bed.
Wear a magnetic bracelet. Drink South Pole magnetised water.
In the case of CFS it is strongly recommended that you sleep on a North Pole orientated magnetic mattress pad.

CIRCULATORY PROBLEMS

Use good quality magnetic innersoles.
Use a magnetic mattress pad.

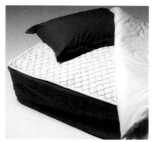

mattress pad

COLDS and FLU

Improve the condition by wearing a small pad over the chest area, and wear a magnetic bracelet.

Drink North Pole magnetised water. If colds and flu are a persistent problem, improve your immune system by using a mattress pad.

COLITIS

Use a small pad over the abdominal area for three to four hours on the first day. Monitor your progress and increase the use of the pad daily. Many patients regularly keep their pad in place all day when the condition flares up. Drink North Pole magnetised water.

CONSTIPATION

Use a small pad over the abdominal area for three to four hours on the first day. Monitor your progress and increase the use of the pad daily. Many patients regularly keep their pad in place all day when the condition persists. Increase your water consumption, and drink North Pole magnetised water.

CRAMPS

Use good quality magnetic innersoles. Use a mattress pad. Increase your water consumption, and drink North Pole magnetised water.

CYSTITIS

Use a small pad over the abdominal area for three to four hours on the first day. Monitor your progress and increase the use of the pad daily. Many patients regularly keep their pad in place all day when the condition persists. Increase your water consumption, and drink North Pole magnetised water.

DEPRESSION

Double blind clinical trials in Japan have shown how helpful it is to sleep on a good quality magnetic mattress pad. Very positive results were seen in over 80% of patients tested.
Wear a magnetic bracelet during the day.

DERMATITIS

Results in treating dermatitis vary greatly from patient to patient, but I would certainly give magnet therapy a try. I suggest the following: Wear a magnetic bracelet on the left hand. Drink North Pole magnetised water and bathe the areas in magnetised water. Magnetise your creams by using the North Pole of a magnet (towards the cream). Use a magnetic mattress pad.

DIABETES

For greatly improved circulation and to offset peripheral neuropathy wear good quality magnetic innersoles. Wear a magnetic bracelet. If possible use a mattress pad or some form of magnetic sleep system. Drink North Pole magnetised water.

powerstrides –
innersoles

EAR ACHE

Apply a 1/2" Neo close to the ear.
For persistent earache consult your doctor.

ECZEMA

Results in treating eczema vary greatly from patient to patient, but I would certainly give magnet therapy a try. I suggest the following: Wear a magnetic bracelet on the left hand. Drink North Pole magnetised water and bathe the areas in magnetised water. Magnetise your creams by using the North Pole of a magnet (towards the cream). Use a magnetic mattress pad.

ENDOMETRIOSIS

Use a small pad over the abdominal area for three to four hours on the first day. Monitor your progress and increase the use of the pad daily. Many patients regularly keep their pad in place all day when the condition flares up. Drink North Pole magnetised water. Use a mattress pad.

LOSS OF ENERGY

Consult your doctor in sudden cases of severe loss of energy.
Move as many electrical appliances from the vicinity of your bed. Use magnetic innersoles. Wear a magnetic bracelet. In severe cases it is recommended that you sleep on a North Pole orientated magnetic mattress pad.

FATIGUE

Move as many electrical appliances from the vicinity of your bed. Use magnetic innersoles. Wear a magnetic bracelet. In severe cases it is recommended that you sleep on a North Pole orientated magnetic mattress pad.

FIBROMYALGIA

Move as many electrical appliances from the vicinity of your bed. Wear a magnetic bracelet. Drink North Pole magnetised water. In the case of FM it is strongly recommended that you sleep on a North Pole orientated magnetic mattress pad. Back this up in the day by applying wraps or neodymium disks to painful sites.

FLATULENCE

Use a small pad over the abdominal area for three to four hours on the first day. Monitor your progress and increase the use of the pad daily. Many patients regularly keep their pad in place all day when the condition flares up. Drink North Pole magnetised water.

FROZEN SHOULDER

Apply one 1" Neo to the back of the shoulder – directly over the 'ouch' area. Leave in place for two or three days to fully eliminate the inflammation. In severe cases a second Neo may be taped to the front of the shoulder.

GALLBLADDER PROBLEMS

Use a small pad over the abdominal area for three to four hours on the first day. Monitor your progress and increase the use of the pad daily. Many patients regularly keep their pad in place all day when the condition flares up. Drink North Pole magnetised water.

GLAUCOMA

Sleep on a North Pole orientated Pillow Pad. Drink magnetised water – and bathe your eyes with North Pole magnetised water daily. Monitor your results with your doctor/optician.

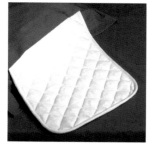

pillow pad

GOUT

The use of a North Pole orientated mattress pad is highly recommended. This will greatly help to remove acidity from the body. When flare-ups occur use a magnetic wrap or 1" Neos over the affected joint. Drink lots of North Pole water.

HAEMORRHOIDS

Sit on a Pillow Pad for at least 3 – 4 hours a day. This period may be increased after a few days. Apply 2 x 1/2" Neos to the base of the coccyx when symptoms are severe. Drink lots of North Pole water.

HEADACHE

Apply 2 x 1/2" Neos to the temples with medical tape. Leave in place until the headache subsides. If you believe your headaches are generated by stress – try taping them to the muscles that run up the back of the neck. This has been found to be very relaxing. For persistent headaches – consult your doctor.

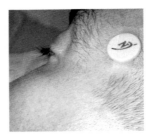

micro neo

HEART CONDITIONS

NEVER USE MAGNET THERAPY IF YOU HAVE A PACEMAKER, DEFIBRILLATOR OR ANY MECHANICAL IMPLANT. MAGNETS WILL AFFECT THE BATTERIES.

Magnet therapy is safe to use if you have had a bypass or if you have metal valves etc. (non-mechanical).
Wearing a good quality magnetic bracelet and innersoles has been seen to be beneficial to improving circulation and general health.

HEEL SPURS

Wearing magnetic innersoles or a 1/2" Neo close to the site has proved to be helpful for the pain, however if you are persistent in using the 1/2" Neo continuously - for two or three months, in many instances – this has eliminated the calcium deposits (bone spur).

INSOMNIA

In non-severe cases a pillow pad will help greatly. Take it with you when you travel. Drink North Pole magnetised water.

In severe and long standing cases, use a good quality mattress pad with magnets of at least 3000 gauss (core). There will need to be a minimum of at least 250 magnets to generate enough relaxation.

IRRITABLE BOWEL SYNDROME

Use a small pad over the abdominal area for three to four hours on the first day. Monitor your progress and increase the use of the pad daily. Many patients regularly keep their pad in place all day when the condition flares up. Drink North Pole magnetised water. Use a mattress pad.

MULTIPLE SCLEROSIS (MS)

Move as many electrical appliances from the vicinity of your bed. Wear a magnetic bracelet. Drink magnetised water. In the case of MS it is strongly recommended that you sleep on a North Pole orientated magnetic mattress pad. Back this up in the day by applying wraps or neodymium disks to painful sites.

KIDNEY PROBLEMS

Drink North Pole magnetised water.
Wear a good quality magnetic bracelet.

MAGNETIC FIELD DEFICIENCY SYNDROME (MFDS)

Move as many electrical appliances from the vicinity of your bed. Wear a magnetic bracelet or innersoles.   Drink North Pole magnetised water. In the case of MFDS it is strongly recommended that you sleep on a North Pole orientated magnetic mattress pad.

MENOPAUSE

Wear a good quality magnetic bracelet. Sleep on a Pillow Pad. Magnetic innersoles will help with the fatigue.

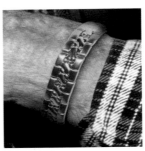

bracelet

MIGRAINE

Apply 2 x 1/2" Neos to the temples with medical tape. Leave in place until the headache subsides. If you believe your headaches are generated by stress – try taping them to the muscles that run up the back of the neck. This has been found to be very relaxing. For persistent headaches – consult your doctor.

NECK PROBLEMS

Use 1/2" Neos taped to the back of the neck. Leave in place until the tension subsides. In severe cases use 1" Neos on the affected area. Sleep on a North Pole magnetic Pillow Pad

NEURITIS

Sleep on a North Pole mattress pad.
Apply a wrap or 1" Neo disks to the affected area during the day. If the loss of sensation is in the legs, wear magnetic innersoles. Drink lots of North Pole water.

OBESITY

There are therapists who claim they can treat obesity with magnet therapy. Certainly sleeping on a mattress pad will encourage the body and organs to work as efficiently as they can, and in some cases that trigger can stimulate increased metabolism.

HOWEVER – the quality and quantity of food that is eaten is in my view, the major factor in weight gain and weight loss.

Drink lots of North Pole water.

OESTEO-ARTHRITIS

Our results in significantly relieving the discomfort and pain associated with arthritis are remarkable. Apply wraps or pads directly over the affected part of the body, as and when it is required. If the arthritis is in several areas of the body, the use of a mattress pad is strongly recommended. Use magnetic innersoles. Double blind studies show that good quality magnet therapy can help over 87% of osteo-arthritis sufferers.

Drink lots of North Pole water.

knee wrap

OSTEOPOROSIS

Move as many electrical appliances from the vicinity of your bed as possible. Wear a magnetic bracelet. Drink North Pole magnetised water. In order to maintain the existing level of bone density and to encourage the body to rebuild itself, we strongly recommended you sleep on a North Pole orientated magnetic mattress pad. Back this up in the day by applying wraps or neodymium disks to painful sites.

PANIC ATTACKS

Sleep on a North Pole magnetic mattress pad or use a pillow pad. Wear a magnetic bracelet.

PARALYSIS

Move as many electrical appliances from the vicinity of your bed. Wear a magnetic bracelet. Drink North Pole magnetised water. In order to encourage the body to see if there is any path back to restoring sensation in the nervous system and possibly to help cells rebuild themselves, we strongly recommended you sleep on a North Pole orientated magnetic mattress pad. If this is not possible, sit on a pillow pad for at least 4 hours during the day.

PERIOD PAIN

Wear a North Pole only - magnetic pad over the tummy area. Make sure the pad is large enough to reach out to the fallopian tubes that sometimes produce the 'dragging' pains.

In severe cases of pain and loss of blood, wearing a magnetic bracelet can help boost the immune system and increase energy levels.

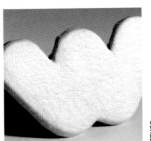

POST-POLIO SYNDROME

Our results in significantly relieving the discomfort and pain associated with many types of Post Polio Symptoms are remarkable. Apply wraps or pads directly over the affected part of the body, as and when it is required. If the pain is in several areas of the body, the use of a mattress pad is strongly recommended. Use magnetic innersoles. Double blind studies show that good quality magnet therapy can help over 84% of sufferers. Drink lots of North Pole water.

PRE-MENSTRUAL SYNDROME (PMT)

Sleep on a magnetic pillow pad.

Wear a North Pole only - magnetic pad over the tummy area. Make sure the pad is large enough to reach out to the fallopian tubes that sometimes produce the 'dragging' pains. In severe cases of pain and loss of blood, wearing a magnetic bracelet can help boost the immune system and increase energy levels.

PSORIASIS

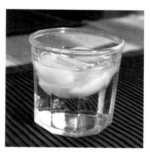

Results in treating psoriasis vary greatly from patient to patient, but I would certainly give magnet therapy a try. I suggest the following: Wear a magnetic bracelet on the left hand. Drink North Pole magnetised water and bathe the areas in magnetised water. Magnetise your creams by using the North Pole of a magnet (towards the cream). Use a magnetic mattress Pad

RHEUMATISM

Our results in significantly relieving the discomfort and pain associated with rheumatism are remarkable. Apply wraps or pads directly over the affected part of the body, as and when it is required. If the pain is in several areas of the body, the use of a mattress pad is strongly recommended. Use magnetic innersoles. Drink lots of North Pole water.

RHUEMATOID ARTHRITIS

This painful condition is not as easy to treat as osteo-arthritis. However, it is certainly worth trying magnet therapy. Double blind studies show we can help over 50% of suffers.

The most effective product would be a good quality North Pole magnetic mattress pad. Wear a good quality bracelet.

Use magnetic innersoles.

RETINITIS PIGMINTOSA

Use a North Pole Pillow and mattress pad.

Treat three times daily with a Magnessage.

I have witnessed remarkable results.

Drink North Pole magnetised water.

SCAR TISSUE

Use 1/2" Neo disks over the scars until the required reduction in damaged tissue is seen. Older scar tissue will require longer treatment of perhaps several months.

SCIATICA

It is best to 'creep' up on this condition, and they way to approach it is with two magnetic pads which can be placed either side of the

lower back or one on the back and one on the back of the knee or calf depending on the route of the pain. Initially keep pads in place for 1 – 2 hours then remove. Increase the period of use as your body becomes accustomed and as you feel the need.

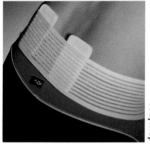

bodywrap

SEXUAL PROBLEMS

It has been found that placing neodymium disks or small pads close to the genitals can stimulate blood flow and relax tissue. I have been told that it is helpful for men to place a disk in their trouser pocket to promote a change in the cell behaviour. Just be careful and DO NOT carry your credit cards in the same pocket. Sleep on a magnetic mattress pad.

SHINGLES

Results in treating shingles vary greatly from patient to patient, but I would certainly give magnet therapy a try. I suggest the following: Use a magnetic mattress pad. Wear a lower back wrap if pain is felt in that area during the day. Drink North Pole magnetised water.

SHOULDER PAIN

Apply 1" Neos to the site.
Wear a good quality magnetic bracelet.

SINUSITIS

Sleep on a magnetic Pillow Pad.

SPRAINS & STRAINS

Use North Pole magnetic wraps or Neodymium disks to the injury. Use the magnets until the injury is healed.

STRESS

Double blind clinical trials in Japan have shown how helpful it is to sleep on a good quality magnetic mattress pad. Very positive results were seen in over 80% of patients tested. Wear a magnetic bracelet during the day.

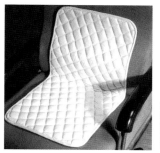

stressbuster

SURGERY

Allow the surgery to settle down for three or four days. Then apply 1/2" Neos gently over the bandaged site. The magnets will encourage the tissue to heal faster and also prevent sever scarring. The Neos will penetrate far enough through the bandage and plasters to affect the tissue beneath.

Do not use magnets following recent heart surgery.

Allow the organ to recover its normal rhythm.

TENNIS ELBOW

Use a good quality elbow wrap or 1" Neos.

TENSION

Wear a good quality magnetic bracelet.

Sleep on a pillow or mattress pad.

TINNITUS

Try using a 1/2" Neo taped behind the ear.

Sleep on a North Pole pillow pad.

TOOTHACHE

Apply a 1/2" Neo to the outside of the affected area.

Sleep on a North Pole pillow pad.

TORN LIGAMENTS & MUSCLES

Use North Pole magnetic wraps or Neodymium disks to the injury.
Use the magnets until the injury is healed.

TRIGEMINAL NEURALGIA

Apply a 1/2" Neo to the outside of the affected area.
Sleep on a North Pole pillow pad.

VARICOS VEINS

Apply a 1/2" Neo to the outside of the affected area.
Monitor the results.
In some cases magnetic innersoles can help with circulatory problems.

WHIPLASH

Sleep on a North Pole pillow pad.
Apply a 1/2" Neo to the outside of the affected area.

WRINKLES

Sleep on a North Pole pillow pad.
Use a mattress pad.
Drink North Pole Magnetised water.

RECOMMENDED THERAPISTS

United Kingdom
Accredited Therapists

Gloria Vergari MCMA
Founder
Norstar Biomagnetics
Unit 4, Pipers Court
Berkshire Drive
Thatcham, RG19 4ER
Tel: 01635 588 888
Email: info@norstarbiomagnetics.com
www.norstarbiomagnetics.com

Lilias Curtin MCMA
30 Delvino Road
Fulham
London SW6 4AD
Tel: 0207 731 4715
Email: locurtin@aol.com

Valerie Dargonne MCMA BSYA (MT)
LCSP (Phys)
8 Sherbourne Road
Hove BN3 8BB
Tel: 01273 421 077
Mobile: 07803 269 418
Email: valdargonne@yahoo.com

Jill Fisher BSc(hons) MIEEE
MCMA
36 Ramsbury Drive
Hungerford, RG17 0SG
Tel: 01488 685422
Email: jill.fisher@ieee.org

Celia Hitchen-Hilsey
Rose Cottage
Knutsford Road
Alderley Edge
Cheshire, SK9 7SS
Tel: 01565 873 753

Jackie Hooper-Moore &
Jenette Atkins
(Equestrian Specialists)
Old Station House
Axbridge
Somerset BS26 2AW
Tel: 01934 733 325

Pat Jones (Humans and
animals).
6 St Marks Avenue
Bilton,
Rugby, CV22 7NP

Sue Kneebone
21 Bowden Hill
Laycock
Chippenham
Tel: 01249 730 379

Alan Moyes MCMA
3 Fleece Cottages
Stanley Downton
Stroud GL10 3QU
Tel: 01453 828 361

Elaine Sawetz
Sports Rehab & Conditioning
Apex Ftness Centre
New Greenham Park
Newbury, RG19 6HN
Tel: 01635 247 351

Barbara – Alexandria's
8 Hilltop Close
Ewloe
Dee Side
Flintshire, CH5 3HA
Tel: 01244 538 178

For more up to date details of accredited magnet therapists in your area please call:

THE BRITISH COMPLEMENTARY MEDICAL ASSOCIATION (BCMA)
PO Box 5122, Bournemouth, BH8 0WG
info@bcma.co.uk
Tel: 01424 438 801

THE COMPLEMENTARY MEDICAL ASSOCIATION (CMA)
Tel: 0208 305 9571   Fax: 0208 305 4888
www.the-cma.org.uk

ACCREDITED COURSE INFORMATION

Norstar Biomagnetics
Unit 4, Pipers Court
Berkshire Drive
Thatcham, RG19 4ER
Tel: 01635 588 888
Email: info@norstarbiomagnetics.com
www.norstarbiomagnetics.com

Lilias Curtin MCMA
30 Delvino Road
Fulham
London SW6 4AD
Tel: 0207 731 4715

Valerie Dargonne MCMA, BSYA (MT), LCSP (Phys)
8 Sherbourne Road
Hove BN3 8BB
Tel: 01273 421 077
Mobile: 07803 269 418
Email: valdargonne@yahoo.com

BOOKS

For a deep understanding of Magnet Therapy; full of up to date information.

> (Our Therapists Favourite)
> Magnet Therapy – The Pain Relief Alternative by Ron Lawrence, M.D., PH.D & Paul Rosch, M.D., F.A.C.P.
> Prima Publishing ISBN 0-7615-1547-X

Easy to read

> The book Book of Magnet Healing by Roger Coghill
> Gaia Books ISBN 1-85675-160-0

In depth understanding of magnetic and electromagnet fields and technology. Of where and where not to locate your electrical plugs and appliances.

> Something in the Air by Roger Coghill
> Coghill Research Laboratories
> Lower Race
> Pontypool, Gwent
> Tel: 01495 763 389

> The Pain Relief Breakthrough by Dr Julian Whitaker, M.D.
> ISBN 0-316-60193-4
> Little, Brown & Company

> Whole Body Healing – by Dr Mark Atkinson MBBS
> Due out Spring 2003
> **a must read – I've seen the draft!**

PRODUCTS WE LIKE

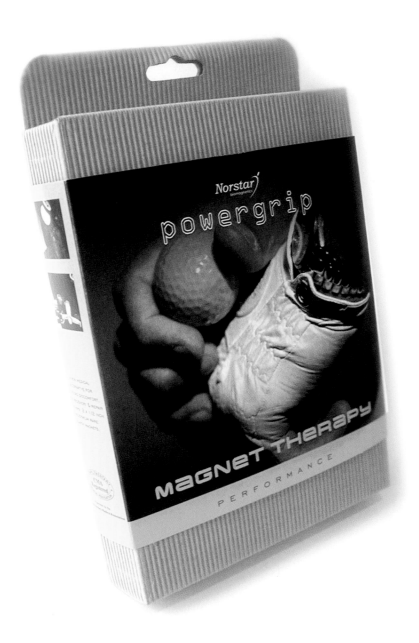

Norstar Biomagnetics International Ltd
Design Consultant – Gloria Vergari MCMA
Full range of high quality products for penetration and results.
Unit 4, Pipers Court
Berkshire Drive
Thatcham, RG19 4ER
Tel: 01635 588 888
Email: info@norstarbiomagnetics.com
www.norstarbiomagnetics.com

Magnotec
Magnetic devices
Tel: 0208 670 5883
Fax: 0208 766 6616

Magne Care USA
800 Indian Springs Road
Chapel Hill
NC 27514
USA
Tel: (919) 789 4778

DOUBLE BLIND STUDIES

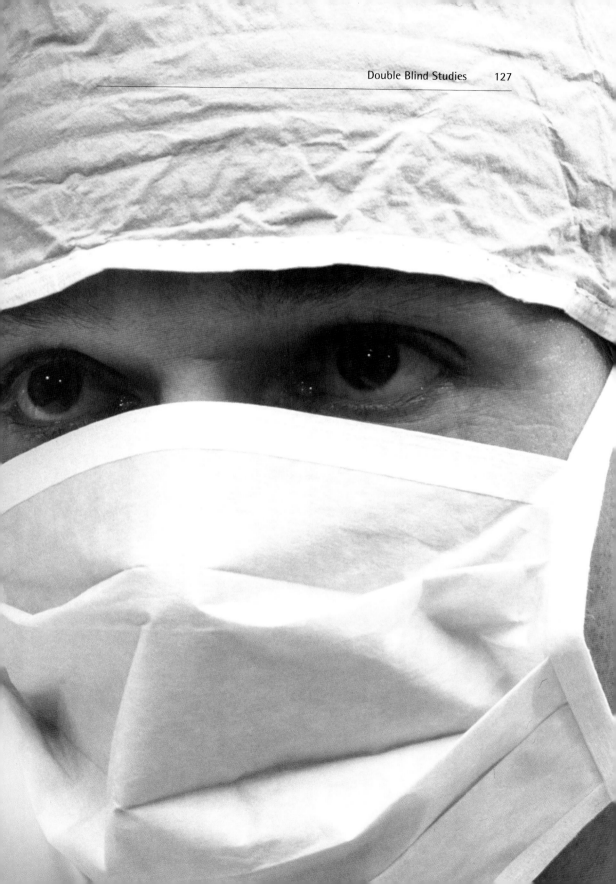

MAGNETIC THERAPY AND ATHLETIC PERFORMANCE

Antonopulos, S. L. (1999, February). Denver Broncos Letter of Testimonial. (Available from Larry Crisp of Preventative Health Care Alliance, 10940 S. Parker Rd., # 426, Parker, CO 80134)

Baker-Price, L. A., & Persinger, M. A. (1996). Weak but complex pulsed magnetic fields may reduce depression following traumatic brain surgery. Perceptual and Motor Skill, 83, 491-498.

Biomagnetic Testimonials. (1999). Magnetic Ideas Inc. Website [On-line]. Available: www.magneticideas.com

Campbell, D. (1997, November 14) New technology relieves chronic pain with magnets. Vanderbilt University Medical Center Reporter, 7, 1,2.

Case Studies and Testimonials. (1999). Quantron Resonance System Website Available: www.quantronic.com

George, M. S., Wasserman, E. M., Kimbrell, T. A., Little, J. T., Williams, W. E., Danielson, A. L . Greenburg, B. D., Hallert, M., & Post, R, M. (1997). Mood improvement following prefrontal magnetic stimulation in patients with depression: A placebo controlled crossover trial. American Journal of Psychiatry, 154, 1752-1756.

Kirkcaldie, M. T. K., Pridmore, S. A., & Pascual-Leone, A. (1997). Transcranial magnetic stimulation as therapy for depression and other disorders. Australian and New Zealand Journal of Psychiatry, 31, 264-272.

Lee, R. C., Canaday, D. J., & Doong, H. (1993). A review of the biological basis for the clinical application of electrical fields in soft-tissue repair. Journal of Burn Care Rehabilitation, 14, 319-335.
Man, D., Man, B., Plosker, H., & Markov, M. (1997). Effect of permanent magnetic field postoperative pain and wound healing in plastic surgery [Online]. Available: www.tectonic.com

Ramey, D. W, (1998). Magnetic and electromagnetic therapy. The Scientific Review of Alternative Medicine, 1, 1-16.

Rogachefsky, R. (1998). Use of tectonic magnet for treatment of hand after gun shot [Online]. Available: www.tectonic.com

Sharrard, W. J. W. (1990). A double-blind trial of pulsed electromagnetic fields for delayed union of tibial fractures. British Journal of Bone Joint Surgery, 72B, 347-355.

Steizinger, C., Yerys, S. Scowcroft, N., Wygand, J., & Otto, R. M, (1999). The effects of repeated magnet treatment on prolonged recovery from exercise induced delayed onset muscle soreness. Medicine and Science in Sports and Exercise Abstracts, 31, 963.

Szor, J. K. (1998). Use of magnetic therapy on an abdominal wound: A case study. Ostomy Wound Manage, 44, 24-29

Valbona, C., Hazelwood, C. F., & Gabor, J. (1997). Response of pain to static magnetic fields in postpolio patients: A double-blind pilot study. Archives of Physical Medicine and Rehabilitation, 78, 1200-1203.